SLOW YOGA

SLOW YOGA
Brian Payne MD PhD

Souvenir Press

First published 2001 by
Souvenir Press Ltd.,
43 Great Russell Street, London WC1B 3PD

ISBN 0 285 63620 0

Printed by Scotprint, Haddington, Scotland

'The wise, for cure, on exercise depend;
God never made his work for man to mend.'
John Dryden
Epistles, to Sir R Howard

Safety

Slow Yoga will help to improve and maintain your health. You should consult your doctor before starting any program of flexibility exercises, including *Slow Yoga,*

- if you are under medical care
- if you have painful joints
- if you have persistent pains in the back, neck, shoulder, arm, wrist, buttock, thigh or calf
- if you have weakness, tingling or numbness anywhere.

Some exercises have health warnings marked with a red triangle:
$\triangle$ *Warning*.
Please be sure to read them.

TABLE OF CONTENTS

Introduction

Why *Slow Yoga*? What is it? And what are its advantages over 'traditional' Yoga?

You probably already know of the health benefits you can gain from traditional Yoga: it calms the mind and reduces stress; it improves flexibility, posture and balance; it strengthens breathing muscles so that you get less breathless on exertion.

Slow Yoga produces all these effects, but also enhances your body health in many other ways. By adopting *Slow Yoga* as your daily exercise plan, you will give yourself the extra benefits of improved muscle tone, increased strength and greater endurance. For *Slow Yoga* is a unique and enjoyable combination of physical exercises used in traditional yoga with slow, sustained muscular tension of the kind used in strength training, but without the need for you to use weights or expensive equipment. And, what is more, you can work at your own pace.

So, *Slow Yoga*

- Gives you all the benefits of Yoga, AND
- Enhances muscle tone. This helps to control your weight by speeding up your basal metabolism
- Increases muscular strength and endurance. These will be invaluable for sports, and you will be providing yourself, at any age, with a reserve that can be called on when you need it
- Augments the strength of muscles around your joints. This will stabilise them and reduce the risk of sprains and falls
- Intensifies the pull of stronger muscles on bone. This will help prevent you from developing osteoporosis (brittle bones)
- Strengthens your body's core muscles and helps you mobilise the joints of your spine. This will decrease your risk of neck and low back pain.

By practising *Slow Yoga* on a daily basis, following the simple exercises in this book, you will increase your general fitness and well-being and, combined with a healthy diet – as with all regular exercise – decrease the risk of diabetes, coronary heart disease, cancer of the colon, fractures and falls, thus giving yourself the prospect of a happy and healthy life.

Follow this easy step-by-step guide and you will see how different your mind and body feel.

Section 1 is about breathing, because of its central role in Yoga. It tells you how breathing works, and shows you how to carry out the five slow breathing exercises that you will use during practice sessions. Slow deep controlled breathing is used to time all movements.

Section 2 is about movement. You will learn how joints and muscles work, how to remedy problems with posture, followed by the main step-by-step *Slow Yoga* exercises. According to the oldest Yoga text, the *Hatha Yoga Pradipika*, Lord Shiva taught 84,000 exercises to his consort Parvani. There are only 25 exercises in this section, in groups of five. Each group moves the spine in a different way, for example, by bending it sideways or twisting it. There are some easier versions for beginners (marked ☺) and harder ones for those who like a challenge (☻). There are special exercises that have been modified for the disabled (♿) and others for later pregnancy (🧎). None of the postures is convoluted and you can work at your own pace.

Illustrations are provided for general guidance, and should not be thought of as ideals to strive for. There is no such thing in *Slow Yoga* as a wrong way of doing exercise – *if it feels good, it is good*. However, there are a few (marked △) where a safer way of carrying out an exercise is suggested, if, for example, you are uncertain of your balance; the same mark is used for the few exercises that are unwise in later pregnancy.

Section 3 tells you about different ways you can choose to practise: how long and how often, and what clothing and equipment you will need. Six daily programs are suggested for you to choose from. You can also devise your own programs by selecting exercises you enjoy from each of the five spinal movement groups. There are exercises you can carry out while shaving or putting on your make up if you are short of time, and six exercises you can do while sitting at work in your office or travelling.

Section 4 tells you about exercise and health, explains the differences between aerobic exercise and the strength training used in *Slow Yoga*, and how a combination of the two can be beneficial, as can a healthy diet. Special exercises are suggested for medical conditions such as osteoarthritis of the knee. And a final chapter shows to how to use *Slow Yoga* to cope with stress.

Slow Yoga is enjoyable and can be done whatever the weather. So why not try it?

SECTION 1: BREATHING

Chapter 1: How breathing works

We do not usually notice that we are breathing in and out. How you think about your breathing and control it is central to *Slow Yoga*. Very slow and deep breathing strengthens the breathing muscles and mobilises the joints. Maximum lung volume is increased and breathing during exertion becomes more efficient, delaying the onset of breathlessness. It helps you relax purposeless muscular tension and it calms a 'whirling' mind. This chapter explains how your muscles and joints are used in breathing work, what can happen if they are not exercised and how their activity is normally controlled without you being aware of it. The last part describes the symptoms to look out for during controlled breathing because they warn you that you are breathing too slow or too fast.

Muscles and joints used when you breathe

The breathing muscles are the diaphragm, the muscles between the ribs, some of the muscles in the neck and the muscles of the abdominal wall.

- The diaphragm is a large thin muscle that stretches across your body dividing the lungs and heart in the chest from the stomach, intestines, liver, spleen and other organs in the abdomen. It is usually described as dome-shaped, but the dome is higher at the front and sides, where it is attached near the lower edge of the rib cage, and lower at the back, where it reaches down to the upper edge of the pelvis. When the muscle contracts the dome shape is flattened, pushing down on the abdominal organs so that the abdominal wall is pushed forward. Air is drawn in and fills mainly the lower parts of the lungs. The pictures show the approximate position of the diaphragm viewed from the side at the end of a breath out (exhalation) and a deep breath in (inhalation).

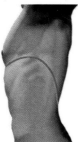 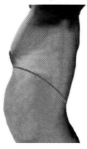

- When the outermost of the three groups of muscles between the ribs (the intercostals) contracts during inhalation the ribs are pulled upwards and outwards, moving like the handle of a bucket when you start to pick it up. Each rib hinges at a joint with the breastbone at the front and with the backbone behind. The pictures show how the handle-like movement increases the volume of the chest. The air drawn in fills the middle and upper parts of the lungs.

- The strap-like accessory breathing muscles in your neck start at the back of your skull and spine and are attached at the top of your chest to the collarbones and the first ribs. When you take a really deep breath they pull the front of the chest forward and upward by up to two and a half inches. The picture shows the accessory muscles that are most easily seen (the sternocleidomastoids). The accessory muscles are used hardly at all during quiet breathing but are called in to play during exertion. The air drawn in fills mainly the tops of your lungs.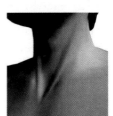

- When breathing out begins, the diaphragm, rib muscles and neck muscles relax and the muscles of the abdominal wall contract. The elastic recoil of the lungs and the chest wall helps the abdominal muscles to expel air, so they do little work during quiet breathing. During forced exhalation, the abdominal muscles are helped by the contraction on the inner layers of muscles between the ribs.

In the slow and deep breathing of *Slow Yoga* your breathing muscles are contracted more strongly and for a longer time than during normal quiet breathing and as a result are greatly strengthened. The next chapter will explain how these movements are carried out.

Effects of lack of exercise on your breathing

When any muscle in your body is not given adequate work it gradually loses bulk and strength so that it can just cope with the small amount it is called on to do. Some wasting affects all the breathing muscles if they are not exercised beyond the level needed for quiet breathing. The most severely affected are those that are used hardly at all in quiet breathing – the accessory neck muscles that raise the front of the chest when there is a great demand for increased ventilation. Couch potatoes can have difficulty with breathing even on slight exertion both because of increased weight due to lack of exercise and because of wasting of all the breathing muscles.

Breathing problems caused by muscle wasting are made worse because the relative immobility it causes affects the joints moved by the breathing muscles. If breathing is always shallow, the joints between the rear of the ribs and the backbone and between the front of the ribs and the breastbone become stiffer. These changes are usually completely reversible with regular exercise. However, in the long-term and particularly in older people chalky material can be deposited in the breastbone joints. The rigidity this causes is not reversible.

The weakness of the breathing muscles and stiffness of the rib joints brought about by lack of exercise do not just reduce the ability of the lungs to cope with increased exertion; they also make it harder for the lungs to deal with other kinds of stress such as congestion due to heart disease and infections such as bronchitis and pneumonia.

Reflex control of breathing

We do not usually notice breathing because automatic reflexes control the muscles. The most sensitive breathing reflex regulates the amount of the soluble gas carbon dioxide that is dissolved in the blood. About one fifth of the air that we breathe in is oxygen. Less oxygen is breathed out than is breathed in because some of it passes from the lungs through the blood stream to the tissues where it is taken up by the cells and used to 'burn' sugars and fats. The energy produced is partly released as heat, but most of it is stored as a high-energy phosphate, adenosine triphosphate (ATP), which is used to power all the chemical reactions necessary for life including muscular activity. The oxygen taken from the air that we breathe in is replaced by an equal volume of carbon dioxide produced by the burning process.

Carbon dioxide is carried from the tissues, dissolved in the blood, to the lungs where it is breathed out. If the amount rises, for example after heavy work when muscle cells have had to produce more energy by burning fuel and have therefore produced more carbon dioxide, the breathing reflex increases the depth and rate of breathing so that the extra carbon dioxide is breathed out.

Deliberate control of breathing

Mental activity can over-ride the normal biochemical reflexes. An increased rate and depth of breathing is common in emotional states such as anxiety. Medical studies have shown that people who are experienced with the kind of slow and deep breathing used in *Slow Yoga* have no significant changes in the amounts of oxygen and carbon dioxide in their blood.

Those who are just beginning the slow breathing used in Yoga sometimes under-breathe. It causes an increase in the carbon dioxide in the blood which produces an intense drive to take a breath. The moment you feel the need, you should stop breathing slowly and take normal breaths until things return to normal. Then try continuing taking deeper slow breaths.

Over-breathing is more common. Fortunately it produces warning symptoms that are easily recognised. It is usually the result of an increase in the depth of breathing with too little slowing of the rate. The amount of carbon dioxide breathed out is increased and the amount of carbon dioxide in the blood reduced. The blood becomes less acid and this affects the nervous system and muscles indirectly by an effect on blood calcium. Symptoms begin with a feeling of light-headedness, followed by numbness and 'pins and needles ' around your mouth and in your fingertips with stiffness of some small muscles in the palms of your hands. Sometimes your chest feels tight and wheezy. If the over-breathing continues, larger muscles go into spasm and eventually convulsions can follow. You should stop the voluntary increase in breathing and let the normal biochemical reflexes take over. All the symptoms will disappear within a few minutes.

During *Slow Yoga* practice you should concentrate on what you are doing and on the sensations produced. One of the reasons is so that you will recognise the earliest warning symptoms of over-breathing and slow your breathing rate down.

Chapter 2: Breathing exercises

The slow breath is used during every *Slow Yoga* exercise, so you should practise it until the movements flow smoothly and naturally. When most people are asked to take a deep breath, their chest expands and their abdomen moves in slightly. In the slow breath the first muscle used is the diaphragm, which pushes the abdominal wall outward (p 3). Breathe right out and see if you can begin to breathe in by pushing your abdomen out. You might find it helpful to lie down comfortably, placing the palm of one hand over the middle of your abdomen and the other on your chest. Practise breathing in and out by pushing your abdomen in and out slowly without using your chest. Once you can do that smoothly, you are ready to learn the *Slow breath*.

When you start practising it is a good idea to stand in front of a mirror so that you can see the movements of your abdomen, chest and neck muscles. A full-length mirror is best, but a dressing table mirror will do.

Initially, breathe in slowly, taking perhaps about five seconds, pause for one or two seconds, take about five seconds breathing out and pause again for one or two seconds. With practice you may find you can comfortably increase these times to eight seconds or more breathing in and out with pauses of three or four seconds. Don't worry if inhalation and exhalation take different times or if your slow breathing rate varies from session to session or from exercise to exercise. Use the slowest rate that you are comfortable with. Always take a normal breath any time you feel the need to do so. Concentrate on what you are feeling and look out for the warning symptoms of breathing too fast which start with a light-headed feeling (p 5).

Slow breath standing

The *Slow breath* strengthens your diaphragm, the muscles between your ribs and the accessory muscles in your neck that pull the rib cage upward at the end of a deep breath in. It mobilises the joints between your ribs and your backbone and between your ribs and your breastbone. It helps to move mucus along your bronchial tubes. Pulling the abdomen in firmly when breathing out strengthens the muscles of your abdominal wall.

1. Stand upright with your hands loosely at your sides and your feet slightly apart so that they are straight below your hips. Your knees should be very slightly bent (not locked back) and you should 'stand tall', lifting the crown of your head. Take a deep normal breath and relax as you breathe out fully through your nose.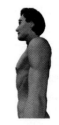

2. Begin the next breath in by letting the front of your abdomen move outwards slowly as the diaphragm pushes downward and forward and the lowest part of your lungs fills with air.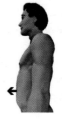

3. Continue inhaling slowly by expanding your chest wall to fill the middle part of your lungs as your ribs move upwards and outwards.

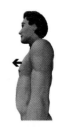

4. Continue a really deep inhalation so that the muscles in the front of your neck can be seen standing out as they fill the upper part of your lungs by pulling the front of your chest upward. Hold your breath for a moment.

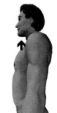

5. Begin breathing out by pulling the centre of your abdominal wall back in slowly and firmly as though you were trying to make your navel touch your backbone. The diaphragm will rise to push air slowly from the lowest part of your lungs. (Your neck muscles should still be standing out.)

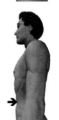

6. Then let your chest wall recoil inwards as air is expelled slowly from the middle parts of your lungs. Keep your abdominal muscles firm.

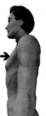

7. Let your neck muscles relax as air is expelled slowly from the upper parts of your lungs. Keep your abdomen firm as you pause again.

Repeat the breath three to eight times, trying to make the movements smooth and continuous.

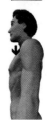

Deep slow breathing helps you to relax purposeless muscular tension and calms your overactive mind, so it can be used during the course of the day before an important meeting or speaking in public, for example. However, don't overdo it – it is a mistake to relax too much before an important occasion because a little anxiety and tension usually adds to performance.

When you are happy with the *Slow breath standing*, practise adding the *Whisper breath*. This involves slightly constricting the voice box while breathing in and out, just as you do when whispering. The sound should be so quiet that someone a few feet away would not hear it. It slightly increases the resistance to the flow of air and so makes the muscles work harder, and it allows you to hear that you are breathing smoothly.

♿ *Disabled*. The *Slow breath* can equally well be done seated but, if possible, sit erect with no back support to allow your ribs and abdomen freedom to move.

Slow breath and stretch

This is the equivalent of a series of good yawns, although breath is taken in through your nose rather than your mouth. It is often used at the beginning of a session, especially a session first thing in the morning. It is an extension of the *Slow breath standing* (p 4). Like the other breathing exercises, it strengthens your diaphragm and chest, neck and abdominal muscles, mobilises the chest joints and helps to clear mucus. In addition, it strengthens your calf and thigh muscles, the muscles that raise the shoulders and the muscles that straighten your elbows because they are held strongly contracted without moving (isometric contractions). It also helps with the return of tissue fluid that has accumulated in your limbs during sleep, and improves balance. Breathe slowly, concentrate on what you are doing and feeling, and don't let your mind wander.

1. Stand upright and tall with your hands loosely at your sides, your feet slightly apart so that they are straight below your hips and your knees very slightly bent. Take a deep breath and relax as you breathe out fully through your nose.

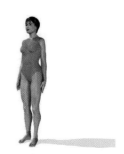

2. Begin the next breath in by letting your abdominal wall push outwards to slowly fill the lowest part of your lungs with air, then expand your chest and continue to inhale really deeply. Immediately after the breath starts, move your arms outwards and upwards in an arc in line with your shoulders, and start to slowly lift your heels off the floor.

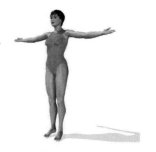

3. Just before the end of the inward breath your arms should be stretching hard above your head with straight elbows, and your heels should be raised as high as you can. Pause for a moment, still reaching high, keeping up the tension in your calves, thighs, shoulders and arms.

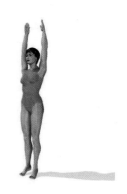

4. Begin to breathe out slowly, pulling your abdomen in firmly, then lower your arms in the same arc and begin to let your heels down.

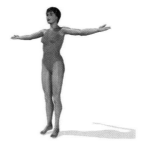

5. Try to have stopped moving and started relaxing you arms and shoulders by the time the breath out is completed. Keep your abdomen firm as you pause.

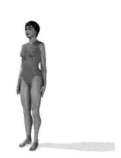

Repeat the breath three to eight times.

☺ *Easier*. If you are uncertain of your balance, instead of standing high on your toes just shift your weight on to the balls of your feet, allowing your heels to stay just in contact with the floor.

☺ *Harder*. If you are confident of your balance, as you begin to inhale in step 2 do not rise on your toes but lift your left foot and rest its arch against the inner side of your right knee with your left knee pointing sideways. Just before the end of the inward breath, with your arms raised above your head, press your palms firmly together as shown in the illustration on the cover of this book. Maintain the tension in your shoulders and arms as you take three or four slow breaths in and out, then slowly lower your arms and leg as you exhale. Repeat standing on the other leg.

♿ *Disabled*. You can do the arm and shoulder part of the *Slow breath and stretch* equally well seated. If possible, sit erect with no back support to allow your ribs and abdomen freedom to move.

Shoulder stand (slow breath upside-down)

It may seem strange that an upside-down posture should be included with breathing exercises. During it the muscles of the shoulder girdle limit chest movement because they are contracted so that your arms can support your body. Most of the work of breathing has to be done by the diaphragm which works much harder than in other positions. With each breath in it has to lift the weight of almost everything in the abdomen, including the liver, spleen and intestines. The shoulder stand is therefore excellent for the strengthening the diaphragm. It also strengthens the muscles that flex your forearms and hands because they are contracted throughout the posture, and it improves balance. It is helpful for clearing mucus from your chest.

△ *Warning*. This posture flexes your neck. If you can touch your chest bone with your chin you need not worry. If you can't, you should place a cushion or pillow under your shoulders which, when fully compressed, is slightly thicker than the gap between your chin and chest.

△ *Warning.* If you have raised blood pressure or glaucoma (raised eye pressure) take medical advice first. If the pressure is well controlled there is unlikely to be a problem. You should also seek medical advice if you have a rather rounded upper back to rule out the possibility that you might have osteoporosis (thinning of the bones).

△ *Warning.* If you are uncertain of your balance, start lying with your feet pointing away from a wall and your head about a foot from it. Then, should you topple backward, the wall will stop you from falling.

As usual, concentrate on what you are doing and feeling; don't let your mind wander.

1. Lie on your back on a mat or folded blanket (a bed, however firm, is not good enough) with support under your shoulders if necessary. Place your arms by your sides with your palms facing down. Take a slow breath in.

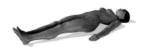

2. As you breathe out, bring your knees up towards your forehead, press down on the floor with your hands and raise your bottom.

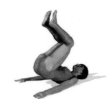

3. As you breathe in, begin to straighten your legs, move your hands to support your bottom and raise your hips. You do not have to force yourself into a straight upside-down position. Stop where your arms and hands need to exert the least pressure to keep your body upright, with your legs still at an angle to the vertical. You can move on to the complete position when you feel ready. Take five to ten slow breaths in this position.

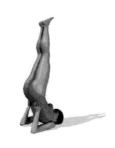

4. When you are ready to come down, breathe normally as you bend your knees and slowly lower them towards your head.

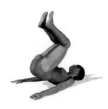

5. Still breathing normally, put your hands back on the floor palms down and slowly lower yourself, feeling each of the bones in your backbone reach the ground as you unroll. Try not to let your head leave the floor. When your bottom has reached the floor, take a slow breath in as you stretch your legs straight up.

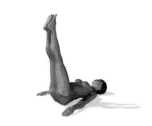

6. Exhale as you slowly lower your legs to the floor with your knees straight.

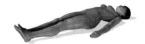

7. Relax and take a few slow breaths. To sit up, slide your feet towards your buttocks until your thighs and lower legs are approximately at right angles. As you exhale hook your hands under your thighs, lift your head and raise your shoulders from the floor, then pull gently on your thighs as you straighten your legs and sit up.

☺ *Harder.* The inner muscles of your thighs can be strengthened while upside-down by letting your legs move slowly apart sideways as you breathe out and bringing them slowly together again as you breathe in.

☺ *Harder.* The muscles of your buttocks and your hamstrings can be strengthened while upside-down by slowly lowering one foot towards the floor over your head as you breathe out and slowly raising it again as you breathe in. Then repeat with the other leg. As usual, try to 'include' the movement within the breath. Begin the movement slightly after the breath out begins, touch the floor (if you can) just before it is complete, begin to raise the leg just after the breath in begins and finish moving just before the breath is complete.

↩ *Pregnancy.* In later pregnancy, instead of using the shoulder stand you can take the pressure off your pelvis and legs by lying with your bottom close to a wall and with your legs resting on it. Press on the wall with your bare feet, slip your hands under your bottom and raise your body as you 'walk' up the wall.

Slow alternate nostril breathing

This is sometimes used at the end of a Yoga session to encourage relaxation. The breathing movements are the same as those of the *Slow breath standing* (p 6). Although this is a relaxation exercise, it provides rather more work for the diaphragm, rib muscles and neck muscles because closing one nostril increases the resistance to breathing in and out, and because the breathing muscles are contracted while the breath is held for a longer time. Do not use this exercise when you have any nasal obstruction, for example a cold.

1. Sit on the floor cross-legged (on a cushion if that is more comfortable) or on a stool or chair. If you use a chair, do not rest against its back. Sit upright with a straight spine.

2. Place the tips of the index and middle fingers of your right hand in the middle of your forehead just above your eyebrows. (If you are left-handed use your left hand and substitute left for right in all that follows.) Your thumb should be resting lightly against your right nostril and your ring and little fingers against the left.

3. Breathe out fully, then close your right nostril with your thumb and begin a slow breath in through the left nostril, taking five to eight seconds.

4. When the breath in is complete, close the left nostril as well with the ring and index fingers and hold your breath for five to eight seconds.

5. Release the right nostril with your thumb and breathe out slowly, taking five to eight seconds.

6. Without pausing, breathe in slowly through the right nostril, hold your breath for five to eight seconds and breathe out slowly through the left nostril.

Repeat the complete cycle five to ten times.

Slow breath lying

This is sometimes used, like *Slow alternate nostril breathing*, at the end of a Yoga session to encourage alert relaxation. The breathing movements are the same as those of the *Slow breath standing* (p 6). Breathe slowly, concentrate on what you are doing and feeling, and don't let your mind wander.

1. Lie on your back on a mat, folded blanket or bath towel or on a firm bed. Support your head with the sort of pillow or cushion that you find comfortable at night.

2. Slide your feet towards your buttocks until your thighs and lower legs are approximately at right angles. Your feet and knees should be a few inches apart and in line with each other.

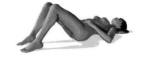

3. Rest your elbows on the floor and place your hands on either side of your abdomen just above the hipbones.

4. Breathe in slowly through the nose by letting your diaphragm push up your abdomen, then expand your chest as described in *Slow breath standing*.

5. Pause for a couple of seconds.

6. As you breathe out slowly, relax and let go of the muscles of your forehead and around your eyes and mouth – sometimes called 'decentralising' the face.

7. On the second breath out relax your neck muscles, letting the nape of your neck move towards the floor.

8. On the third breath out relax your shoulder muscles and let both shoulders fall back towards the floor.

9. Continue working down both arms and then your chest, abdomen, buttocks and legs until your whole body feels heavy and is pressing into the floor.

If you like you can begin with the feet, then the calves, thighs, buttocks, abdomen and chest, then the fingers, forearms, upper arms, shoulders, neck and face.

↩ *Pregnancy.* You can modify *Slow breath lying* to help relieve swelling of the ankles and leg veins as the baby grows: rest your feet on a chair or against a wall instead of on the floor, with your knees bent at right angles.

↩ *Pregnancy.* If you find lying on your back is uncomfortable or unpleasant because of pressure from the baby, the *Slow breath lying* can be done lying on your side. Place a pillow under your head and another beside your waist to rest your arm and abdomen on, and perhaps a third pillow or cushion to support your bent leg.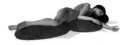

Do not get up too suddenly after this period of alert relaxation because you may become faint or giddy. As you exhale, hook your hands under your thighs, move your head forward on to your chest, raise your shoulders from the floor and sit up slowly as you straighten your legs. Take a minute or two before standing. (And don't drive for another 15 minutes or so – a driver who is too relaxed is not good for road safety!)

When you come to design your own practice programs (p 56) it is a good plan to include two breathing exercises, one at the beginning and one at the end. On a bad day, when you really do not have time for even a short session of *Slow Yoga*, you will find that the day goes better if you start it with the *Slow breath and stretch* rather than just a yawn.

SECTION 2: MOVING

Chapter 3: How your joints and muscles work

The bones, joints, muscles and nerves involved in movement need a healthy flexible spine. This chapter explains the importance of keeping your spine and limb joints mobile, the effects of lack of exercise and poor posture, and the benefits of *Slow Yoga* strength training.

Spinal joints

Your spinal column is made of 34 vertebral bones stacked on top of one another, separated by vertebral discs. The spine curves forward in the neck region, backward in the chest region, forward again in the small of back (the lumbar region) and backward at the bottom of the spine.

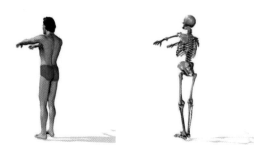

The discs between the vertebrae have a tough flexible outer shell and a soft jelly-like centre. They are elastic with a consistency like an India rubber eraser, although they are slower to regain their shape after being distorted. They act as shock absorbers, and allow a small amount of bending and twisting between adjacent vertebrae. They gradually lose water and become thinner during activity and regain it during rest, so that we are taller first thing in the morning than when we go to bed.

There are facet joints between the vertebrae in addition to the discs. The pictures show top and side views of a lumbar vertebra with, ringed in red, two bony processes pointing upwards and facing inwards, and two pointing downwards and facing outwards. They have cartilage-lined facets which are smooth and slippery when wet.

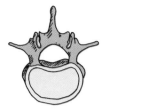 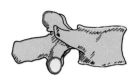

The facets on each vertebra form four joints, two with the facets on the vertebra above and two with those on the vertebra below.

This picture shows how the facet joints fit together. The red line around the cartilage represents a membrane that produces a viscous slippery lubricating fluid rather like egg white, the synovial fluid. The cartilage-covered surfaces glide on each other, sliding like the joints between the jawbone and the skull during chewing.

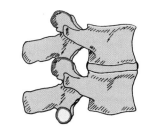

The synovial fluid contains plasma filtered from the blood. This is absorbed into the cartilage when the joint is resting, and is squeezed out again during activity when the surfaces are pressed together. In this way nutrients are supplied to the cartilage cells and waste materials are removed. All the joints in our limbs have a similar structure.

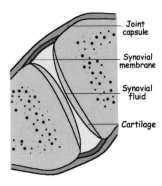

Effects of inadequate joint movement

If a joint is used regularly and taken through its full range of movement (by Yoga exercises for example) its synovial membrane is thick, has a rich blood supply and is thrown into folds so that it has a large surface area. Recent research has shown that when a joint is little used it has a smaller blood supply, the synovial membrane thins, it loses most of its folds and the production of synovial fluid is reduced. The compression and decompression of the joint that nourishes the cartilage cells during normal activity is also reduced. As a result of these changes caused by limited movement, joints can become very stiff. Of the movements of the spine, twisting is usually the first to lose flexibility because of inactivity. Stiff joints can easily be injured if they are made to move through an unaccustomed range.

Injury of stiff spinal facet joints is one cause of neck, shoulder or low back pain. The spinal nerves (marked *0* in the picture) and their blood vessels emerge from the spinal canal between the vertebrae through 'windows' on each side between the vertebral discs in front and the facet joints behind. You can see how an injured, swollen facet joint protruding forward could press on a nerve just like a 'slipped' disc protruding backward, causing pain or numbness and sometimes muscle weakness.

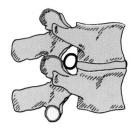

Muscles that move the spine

Most of the core muscles that bend and twist your spine and help to maintain a normal posture are attached to the vertebrae. Muscles that are collectively called the erector spinae lie behind the backbone in the grooves on each side of the vertebrae along its whole length. The picture shows a cross-section through the lumbar region of the spine.

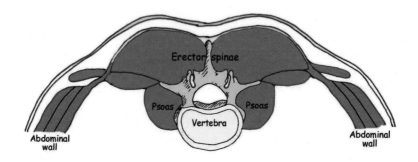

The psoas muscles are attached to your backbone in the lumbar region and run down through your groin to attach to the inner side of the femur (thigh bone) just below the hip joint. The prevertebral muscles lie in a similar position in your neck. All these core muscles are strengthened by *Slow Yoga* exercises.

Some muscles that do not run alongside your spine help to bend it forward and sideways. The breathing muscles in your neck that are attached to your collarbone and the top of your rib cage (p 4) help to bend your neck forward. The three layers of muscle that make up the side walls of your abdomen are attached to the erector spinae muscles on each side at the back and to the rectus muscles ('six pack') at the front, and help with bending and twisting movements. The rectus muscles that make up the front wall of your abdomen are attached to the bottom of your rib cage and the top of the pubic bone. They help to bend the lumbar region forward and stop your abdomen ballooning out when the side muscles contract. These muscles are strengthened by *Slow Yoga* breathing exercises as well as by the general exercises.

Your trunk is converted into a rigid pillar by holding your breath and contracting all the core spinal and abdominal muscles. The trunk can then provide leverage for the arm and leg muscles to lift, push or pull a heavy weight. When lifting, it is best to start from a squatting position. Lifting heavy objects by bending forward with a curved back can damage the ligaments, joints and muscles of your lower back because the hamstrings normally begin to lift the spine before the back muscles, the erector spinae, contract. Localised spasm of damaged muscle and the swelling of damaged facet joints can then squeeze spinal nerves and cause low back pain.

Effects of inadequate muscular activity

The health of your muscles depends on regular physical activity. Muscles that are not exercised adequately gradually lose bulk and strength. If you have ever had a joint immobilised in a plaster cast because of a fracture you will remember how weak the muscles that move the joint felt when the plaster was removed, and that they took several days to regain full strength. It has been estimated that completely immobilized muscles lose 5% of their strength a day.

General lack of strength of your spinal muscles can lead to poor posture and its consequences, and can also increase the risk of unsteadiness and falls. Many people become so sedentary as they get older that their muscles atrophy tremendously and they become frail. Muscle training can often more than double their strength.

Effects of poor posture

Normal posture is maintained by reflex messages sent to the spinal cord from muscles, joints, tendons and ligaments about their tension and position. The muscles receive a return message from the spinal cord telling them how to contract sufficiently to maintain a steady postural tone and how to respond to small changes to maintain a steady position. When we want to move, messages travel from the brain down the spinal cord to nerve cells that supply the muscles we need to contract. At the same time that the nerve cells instruct that group of muscles to contract, a message goes to the opposing group of muscles telling them to relax their normal reflex postural tone.

Problems can arise when your muscles are stretched not by a slow deliberate voluntary movement but by the momentum that follows a sudden movement. For example, if you bounce down hard to touch your toes, the hamstring muscles in the back of the thighs are pulled on while they are still maintaining a normal postural contraction, and muscle fibres, ligaments and even tendons can be torn. This is probably the commonest sort of sports injury. One of the reasons for recommending *Slow Yoga* is that it is safe from the risks of sprains, strains and tears.

The normal postural reflex can be affected by subconscious messages from the higher centres. The drooping shoulders and bent back of someone with depression illustrates this well, and can cause neck and shoulder pains. The normal reflex can also be altered by a constant pull, for example from the increased abdominal weight of pregnancy or obesity. There is a tendency to counteract the weight by leaning back, with an increased curve in the small of your back, often causing low back pain. Similarly, if a hip or knee joint is painful, the reflex posture of your spine may be altered so that sideways bends reduce pressure on the affected side.

If an abnormal posture becomes habitual, the reflexes can become reset to work in that position, causing lengthening or shortening of parts of the capsules of the spinal facet joints and discs and of the muscles that move them, and narrowing the spinal widows between the vertebrae. The good news is that if a correct posture is maintained by thinking about how you stand and sit, in the long run that, too, will become an automatic reflex. Correct posture keeps the spinal windows wide open so that there is no pressure on the nerves and blood vessels that pass through them. The simple message is to think tall, stand tall, sit tall.

In the normal erect posture your head is directly above your feet, looking forward and held high. The forward curves of your spine at the nape of your neck and in the lumbar region, and the backward curves of your chest and buttocks are not exaggerated. Your shoulders are relaxed, not pulled back, and the knees are very slightly bent, not locked. During walking or running, the weight of your head and shoulders is cushioned by the elasticity of the discs and by slight increases of the backward and forward curvatures of the spine. This cushioning also takes place when a weight is held in the hands. All the joints between the vertebrae are at about their midpoint so that they are able to bend a roughly equal distance forward and backward. The spinal nerve windows between the vertebrae are in their most open position.

In the swayback posture the forward curve in the lumbar region is greatly exaggerated, causing the spine in the chest region and the buttocks to be thrust backward. This causes no problems if it is only a transient position. However, because the lumbar curvature is at the extreme limit of normal, if it is maintained the curve becomes even more exaggerated when a downward load is applied by walking, running or carrying a weight. This narrows the windows through which the spinal nerves emerge and is a potential cause of back discomfort or pain.

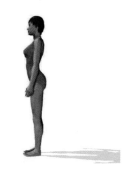

Scoliosis (side-to side bending of the spine) is usually caused by disease, often as a result of a painful hip or knee joint on one side. Taking one's weight on one leg for prolonged periods can produce discomfort. If the weight is taken on the left leg, the pelvis tips down to the right, the spine in the lumbar region becomes concave to the left, the chest region concave to the right with one shoulder higher than the other, and the neck region concave to the right. A similar effect can be produced by sitting awkwardly, for example on a couch working on a coffee table for prolonged periods. The spinal nerve windows are narrowed on one side or the other along the whole spine, producing discomfort or pain almost anywhere.

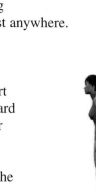

A stooped posture is by far the most common. The pelvis is tipped so that the lumbar curve is flattened. The backward curvature of the spine in the upper part of the chest region is exaggerated and so is the forward curvature in the neck region. They are both held near the extreme of normal. A downward load caused by walking, running or particularly carrying a heavy weight exaggerates these upper curves and narrows the spinal nerve windows, potentially producing neck, shoulder or arm discomfort or pain. Similar symptoms can result from sitting with a curved back looking down at a desk or a badly placed computer screen for long periods.

You can find out whether you habitually have a stooped posture quite simply. The ligaments that run down the spine will have tended to shorten in front of the vertebrae in the upper part of the chest and behind the vertebrae in the neck, and the discs will have become more wedge-shaped. The test is to stand with your back against a wall, slide your feet forward until the small of your back touches the wall and your legs are at about 45° to the floor. As you take a slow breath

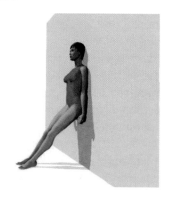

in, gently attempt to push your head back against the wall, keeping your chin tucked in. If you can do this easily, you have no permanent problem.

△ *Warning.* Don't do this if you are over 40 and have an obviously rounded upper back. Seek medical advice to rule out the possibility of osteoporosis (thinning of the bones).

If it causes any discomfort, you can improve things by holding the position that just starts to feel uncomfortable as you pause at the end of the slow breath in. Let your head come forward as you breathe out and repeat for three to six slow breaths. The straightening of the spine in the chest region can be helped as you breathe in by stretching your arms out sideways and bending your elbows at right angles so that the backs of your hands are against the wall opposite your head. If this is repeated daily it will gradually stretch the shortened ligaments and allow the discs to regain their shape.

Practising the *Slow breath lying* (p 12) daily will also help to straighten and lengthen your spine. In addition, your muscle tone will improve and help you achieve a normal posture if you adopt a regular *Slow Yoga* exercise plan to strengthen your core muscles and if you always try to think tall, sit tall and stand tall.

Benefits of Slow Yoga strength training

Most kinds of exercise prevent muscle wasting and joint stiffness. Traditional Yoga physical practice improves flexibility, posture and balance. *Slow Yoga* incorporates an element of strength training to improve lung function, muscle tone, strength and endurance as well.

The strength training used in *Slow Yoga* consists of loading muscles so that they use one half to two thirds of their maximum force for five to ten seconds at a time. It has been shown that maximum strength develops with five or so repetitions of this kind five days a week.

We usually think of muscular contraction as a shortening and widening of muscle as the name suggests, like the contraction seen when we bend our elbow to demonstrate the size of our biceps muscle. When a heavy object is lifted from a chair and placed on a table, the arm, shoulder and back muscles contract and shorten. However, when the weight is lifted from the table and replaced on the chair, the muscles contract (pull) while they are lengthening. If the weight is held stationary in the half way position, the muscles are contracted but are neither shortening nor lengthening, an isometric contraction. Clearly, isometric contractions are easily sustained for five to ten seconds at a time, but shortening or lengthening movements during an exercise last as long as five to ten seconds only if they are done slowly. In *Slow Yoga,* muscles are loaded with the weight of the head, trunk or limbs instead of with the resistance of external weights or springs, and movements are made slowly. Sometimes one group of muscles is used to push against another in an isometric contraction. Isometric contractions are continued during the pauses at the end of inspiration and expiration.

How do resistance exercises increase strength? A man with underdeveloped muscles can increase their size by 50% with a few months training. For many years it was assumed that strength gain was entirely the result of increased muscle size. It is certainly a factor. The increase in size is large in men and small in women because of the influence of the male sex hormone testosterone.

With no noticeable increase in the size of her muscles, a woman using the same exercise program as a man can gain the same amount of strength. There is now good evidence that the nervous system is involved in the strength gain from resistance training. The individual fibres that make up muscle contract in response to messages from the spinal nerves, but not all the fibres in a muscle contract at the same time. Training increases the number of fibres that respond to a given stimulus, thus increasing strength without necessarily increasing muscle size. Reports of superhuman feats of strength during moments of intense psychological stress are probably accounted for by immense nervous stimulation of muscle making all the fibres contract simultaneously.

Strength training is of value to people of all ages, from the young to the very old. The elderly benefit because the increased strength of muscles around joints stabilises them and helps to reduce the risk of sprains and falls. Strength training decreases the risk of osteoporosis and has been shown to reverse the syndrome of physical frailty.

The young and fit can benefit in a number of ways. *Slow Yoga* increases the strength of your breathing muscles and mobility of the rib joints, so making it easier to respond to the demands of severe exertion. 'Second wind' is reached earlier and 'stitch' is uncommon. Strength training also increases endurance – the ability to repeat the same muscle actions for a long time. This is a rather unexpected consequence of training that involves only short periods of exertion. The increased endurance is due to increased muscle enzyme activity, increased high-energy phosphate compounds including ATP providing increased energy stores, and increased muscle glycogen and triglyceride providing fuel stores. This increased capacity for both sustained exertion and for short bursts of hard work is valuable to those who take part in all kinds of sport.

In contrast, aerobic exercises like walking, jogging and running also increase endurance, but because they provide little resistance to muscle action they result in little or no increase in strength.

Taking part in a sport does not increase your capacity for it. Overload – working against loads larger than those usually encountered – is necessary for development, and should form part of any good training program. Yoga-type flexibility movements are often used for warming-up before starting a sporting activity and for 'warming-down' afterwards. *Slow Yoga* can be used as an intrinsic part of a training program to provide strength overload and so increase both your strength and endurance.

Principles of Slow Yoga

The 25 main exercises are described in the next five chapters, and choosing an exercise program is discussed in the following Section (p 53). The exercises should be practised according to the following principles:

1. Synchronise your movements with slow breathing:
   - Inhale slowly starting with the diaphragm, then the chest muscles, then the neck muscles
   - Pause of a few seconds in full inspiration
   - Exhale slowly with the stomach muscles, then relax the chest, then the neck muscles
   - Pause for a few seconds in full exhalation.

2. Carry out movements slowly and the hold muscles tense when not moving:
   - Start to move after you start inhaling
   - Slowly take the movement to a comfortable limit and contract the muscles firmly before completing the inhalation
   - Keep the muscles tense during the pause after full inspiration
   - Begin the next slow movement just after releasing the tension and starting exhalation
   - Contract the muscles, including the abdominal muscles, firmly during the pause after full exhalation.

3. Concentrate on what you are doing and feeling when you are exercising; try not to let thoughts about the past or the future intrude. Full awareness will allow you to push your limits comfortably without the risk of pain or soft tissue injury.

Chapter 4: Backward bends

Unlike the other exercises in this Section, these bend the spine in only one direction. It is pleasant to follow them with a 'counterpose' – a short relaxing forward bend.

Back arch standing

This is a good exercise for improving balance. It mobilises the joints of your upper spine and the shoulders in extension. It strengthens the erector spinae muscles of your back and the flexor and extensor muscles of your thighs and lower legs. It puts considerable strain on your hips and knees, so if you have trouble with those joints carry it out without bending your knee. Breathe slowly, concentrate on what you are doing and feeling, and don't let your mind wander.

1. Stand facing forward with your feet two to three feet apart, so that you can feel that the muscles on the inner sides of your thighs are being gently stretched.

2. Turn your left foot on its heel until it is pointing to the left. Lift your right heel and swivel it backward on the ball of the foot until it is at 45 degrees, as shown in the picture. Take a slow breath in as you turn to the left, raising your arms and stretching them sideways as strongly as you can.

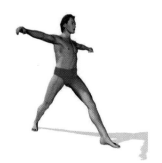

3. As you breathe out, drop downward by bending your left knee until your thigh is nearly horizontal. Swing your arms together and stretch them forward firmly. As usual, try to 'include' the movement within the breath.

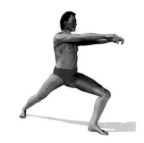

4. As you begin a slow inhalation, slowly stretch both arms high above your head, look upward and then firmly pull your arms, head and shoulders backward as far and as strongly as is comfortable. Hold this position for a few seconds at the end of inhalation.

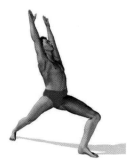

5. As you breathe out, straighten your head and spine, lower your arms, relax your shoulders, straighten your knee and look forward.

Do three to six complete repetitions to the left from step 2, then change the position of your feet and repeat on the right.

Counterpose: With your legs still apart, turn both feet forward, raise your arms high above your head as you take a slow breath in. Sweep your arms down towards the floor as you exhale and bend your trunk forward. Let your head hang down. Take three or four normal breaths in this position. Concentrate on letting go of tension in your hamstrings, buttocks and back.

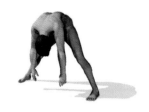

☺ *Harder.* After you have held the back arch and begin to breathe out in step 4, straighten your knee, slowly bend forward and reach for the floor near your feet with your hands. Hold for a few seconds, and then take a slow breath in as you unfold, straighten your spine and look forward.

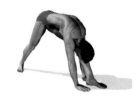

♿ *Disabled.* The arm and shoulder movements in steps two, three and four can be carried out seated on the front edge of a stool or chair.

Back arch lying

This exercise is for the middle and lower end of the spine. It mobilises the hips and vertebral facet joints in extension and strengthens the hamstrings, the gluteal muscles in the buttocks and the erector spinae muscles of the back.

1. Lie on your back with your arms by your sides. Draw your feet towards your buttocks, raising your knees, until the small of your back touches the floor. Take a slow breath in.

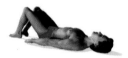

2. As you begin to exhale and tighten your abdominal muscles, tilt the front of your pelvis towards your head and slowly raise your buttocks as high as you can from the floor. You will feel your head slide back a little along the floor.

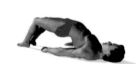

3. Hold this bridge position as you take a second slow inhalation, keeping your hamstrings and the muscles of your back and buttocks tight. If you can, shuffle your feet a few inches nearer your head.

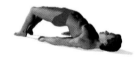

4. As you breathe out, again tilt your pelvis towards your head as you lower yourself to the floor. Your spine should reach the floor from above downwards: the chest region first, then the upper lumbar, lower lumbar and pelvis. Your head will slide forward.

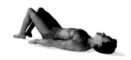

Inhale slowly, and then begin again from step 2 above. Repeat three to six times.

Counterpose: Inhale slowly as you raise your bent legs and take hold of your knees, keeping you arms straight. Exhale slowly as you pull your knees firmly towards your chest. Inhale as you relax your arms again. Repeat two or three times and then rest with your feet on the floor.

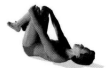

☺ *Easier.* If you find it difficult to hold the bridge position for a full slow breath, raise your buttocks as you breathe in and return to the floor as you breathe out.

☺ *Harder.* In step 2, as you exhale while slowly raising your buttocks as high as you can from the floor, also slowly raise your right leg until it is pointing straight up. Hold the muscles tense as you pause. During exhalation, bend your knee and lower your right foot next to your left foot on the floor. Repeat an equal number of times on each side.

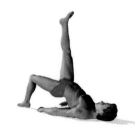

Chest and neck arch prone

This exercise mobilises the vertebral joints of the upper spine in extension. It provides stronger strength training for the erector spinae in the chest and nape of the neck than the *Back arch standing* because the muscles have to lift the weight of the head and part of the chest. It is followed by a relaxing forward bend.

1. Lie on your stomach with your arms by your sides, palms up. Take a slow breath in and hold it for a few seconds.

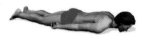

2. As you begin to breathe out, raise your head and shoulders from the floor and look forward and upward as far as is comfortable.

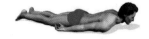

3. Hold the position while you take a second slow inhalation, and pause for a few seconds.

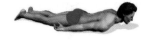

4. As you breathe out, slowly lower your head and shoulders to the floor.

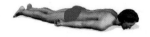

Repeat three to six times. Don't worry if your chin rises only an inch or so from the floor at first – the muscles will soon strengthen and the spine become more flexible.

Counterpose: Kneel upright as you take a slow breath in. Sit back on your heels as you begin to breathe out, bend forward and slowly lower your head to the floor, sweeping your arms back so that they lie alongside your legs, palms facing upwards. Take half a dozen normal breaths in this position as you let go of tension in your back, neck and shoulders.

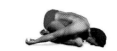

☺ *Easier*. If you have difficulty raising your head and shoulders, start with your arms resting on the floor in front of you with the elbows bent. Press gently downward on the floor with your hands to start to raise your head and shoulders. Remember that the objective is to pull your head up with your back and neck muscles, not to push it up with your arms. Do not go beyond a comfortable position.

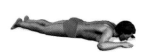

☹ *Harder*. As you raise your head and shoulders from the floor, swing your arms outwards and forward and hold them raised off the floor in front of your head until you start to breathe out. Then bring them back until they are again alongside your body by the time your head and shoulders reach the floor. This provides excellent strength training for the shoulder and back muscles.

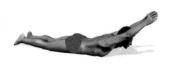

△ *Warning in pregnancy.* The exercise exerts considerable pressure on the abdomen and is inadvisable after very early pregnancy.

Leg and lumbar arch prone

This exercise mobilises the joints of your lower spine and your hip joints in extension. It provides more strength training than the *Back arch lying* for the erector spinae in the lower part of your back and for your buttock and calf muscles because the whole weight of the lower limbs is supported. It is followed by a relaxing forward bend.

1. Lie on your stomach with your arms by sides, your hands forming loose fists, thumbs against the floor. Take a slow breath in.

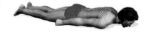

2. As you exhale, slowly raise both your feet and legs (and your pelvis if you are able to) from the floor as high as you can comfortably, helped by firm downward pressure from your fists. Hold this position while you take a slow breath in.

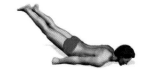

3. Slowly lower your legs to the floor as you exhale.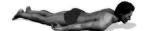

Repeat three to six times.

Counterpose: Use the kneeling posture described above.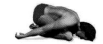

☺ *Easier*. Raise only one leg at a time. Perform equally on each side.

☻ *Harder*. As you raise your feet and legs from the floor, swing your arms outwards and forwards and hold them raised off the floor in front of your head until you start to breathe out. Then bring them back until they are again alongside your body by the time your legs reach the floor. This provides excellent strength training for the muscles of the shoulder and back.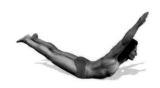

△ *Warning in pregnancy*. This exercise exerts considerable pressure on the abdomen and is inadvisable after very early pregnancy.

Back arch prone

In this exercise the arm and shoulder muscles pull against the leg and hip muscles to arch the spine backward. The vertebral and hip joints are mobilised. It is very important to concentrate on what you are doing, to pull slowly and gently and to slacken the pull at the first sensation of discomfort to avoid hyperextending the spine.

1. Lie on your stomach with your arms by sides, palms facing upward. Take a slow breath in.

2. As you inhale, reach backward with both hands, raise your feet and hold on to your ankles. You may find that the easiest way to do this is to slide your knees apart on the floor as you raise your feet and to begin to slide your legs together when you have hold of your ankles. Pause for a moment.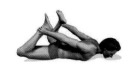

3. Exhaling slowly, raise your head and chest and pull your ankles upward and backward until you are resting on the centre of your trunk. Look forward. Take a slow breath in as you hold that position, keeping up the tension.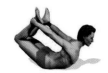

4. As you exhale slowly, slacken the pull and let your chest and thighs return to the floor, keeping hold of your ankles.

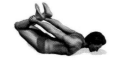

Repeat from step 3 three to six times.

Counterpose: Use the kneeling posture described above. You can use this restful posture to recover after any of the exercises described later in the book that you find strenuous.

△ *Warning in pregnancy.* This exercise exerts considerable pressure on the abdomen and is inadvisable after very early pregnancy.

Chapter 5: Forward and backward bends

Forward and backward bend standing

This exercise mobilises your vertebral joints in flexion and extension and takes your shoulder joints through a wide range of movement. It supplements work for the spinal flexor and extensor muscles with strength training for all the muscles around your shoulders. Breathe slowly, concentrate on what you are doing and feeling, and don't let your mind wander.

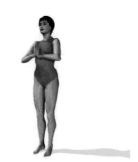

1. Stand with your feet a couple of inches apart and take a slow breath in. As you begin to breathe out, bring your hands together in front of your chest, fingers pointing upward. Press your palms firmly together, bending the wrists back as far as is comfortable. Keep up the pressure as you pause for a few seconds.

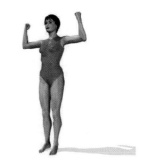

2. As you begin the next slow inhalation, raise your arms sideways, elbows bent at right angles and pulled back, make fists and rotate them firmly so your knuckles face as far to the front as possible. Keep you chin tucked in. Hold your breath for a few seconds, keeping up the tension in your biceps and other arm muscles.

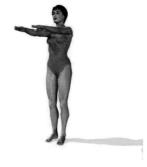

3. As you exhale, push your arms straight out in front of you so that your shoulders are pulled forward and the muscles in the front of your chest (the pectorals) stand out. Keep up the tension as you pause.

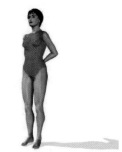

4. During the next slow inhalation, move your hands behind your back at the level of your waist, interlock your fingers and press your hands firmly together. (Do not be alarmed by cracking noises from the shoulder joints.) Keep up the pressure as you hold the inhalation for a few seconds.

5. During exhalation move your head and shoulders backward, straighten your elbows and push your interlocked hands downwards as firmly as you can to pull on the spine. Hold for a few seconds. (You can pause here and take two or three normal breaths if you wish, keeping up the pull.)

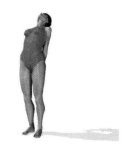

6. As you take a slow breath in, raise your straightened arms as high as you can behind you and begin to bend your head forward. (If you like, at this stage you can turn your interlocked hands over so that the palms face away from you.)

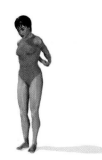

7. As you slowly exhale, roll your spine forward and downward as far as is comfortable, keeping your arms straight, until they are stretched above you. Take two or three normal breaths in this position, concentrating on the sensations in your buttocks and hamstrings, and letting go of any tension with each exhalation.

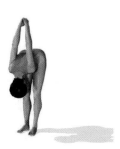

8. When you are ready, take a slow breath in and slowly 'unroll' your spine to stand upright with your hands by your sides.

Do two to four complete repetitions.

♿ *Disabled.* If you are able to sit on a stool you can lower your interlocked hands behind your back at step 5. At step 7, simply bend forward as far as is comfortable.

🤰 *Pregnancy.* In later pregnancy start with your feet apart so that you can accommodate your abdomen when you bend forward.

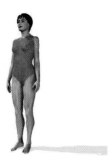

Forward and backward bend on hands and knees

These bends mobilise all the joints of your spine in flexion and extension, and provide strength training for a surprisingly wide range of muscles. When your back is hollowed, all of the erector spinae muscles and some of the shoulder girdle muscles are under tension. When your back is arched upward, the muscles contracted include those of the pelvic floor, the psoas, the abdominal muscles and the prevertebral muscles.

1. Kneel on all fours with your knees slightly apart and your hands flat on the floor below your shoulders.

2. As you take a slow breath in, slowly raise your head to look forward and upward as far as is comfortable, hollowing your back downward. Keep up the tension as you pause for a few seconds.

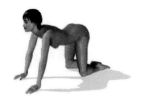

3. As you contract your abdominal muscles at the beginning of breathing out, arch your back upward, pull your head downward and tuck your chin in to your chest, tilt your pelvis forward to 'tuck in your tail' and firmly tighten your pelvic floor – the muscles that are used to prevent accidents when one has diarrhoea or a full bladder and that contract during orgasm. Keep up the tension as you pause for a few seconds.

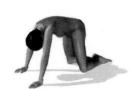

4. From this position, start a slow inhalation, slowly hollow your back and start again from step 2.

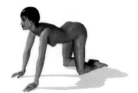

Repeat these movements three to six times.

☺ *Easier.* If you have trouble kneeling, start from a standing position. Then lean forward and place your hands on a bed or the seat of a chair.

☺ *Harder.* As you breathe in and hollow your back downward, extend your right arm straight in front of you and your left leg straight behind you. As you breathe out and arch your back upward, return them to the floor. Repeat an equal number of times on each side.

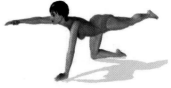

Forward and backward bend on hands and feet

In this exercise the hands and feet support the body throughout, while the spine is held in both backward and forward bends. It mobilises all the joints of the spine and the disc capsules, and strengthens the spinal flexors and extensors and the muscles of the shoulders, arms, back, buttocks and legs.

1. Kneel on the floor, sit back on your feet and take a slow breath in.

2. As you begin to breathe out, bend forward so that your head is close to or on the ground and place your hands on the ground in front of you at about shoulder width apart.

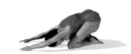

3. As you inhale slowly, come up on to your hands and knees. As you start to exhale, tuck your toes under, straighten your legs, and slowly drop your pelvis forward and downward so that your back is arched, you are looking forward and your weight is carried on your hands and feet with your knees off the ground. Slowly inhale in this position.

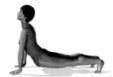

4. As you begin the next exhalation, slowly swing your pelvis backward and upward and your head backward and downward so that you are looking at your feet. Straighten your legs as far as you can without discomfort. Inhale and pause in this position.

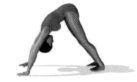

5. As you exhale, slowly drop your pelvis forward and downward and look forward. Inhale in this position and pause.

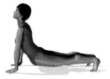

Repeat the upward and downward movements (steps 4 and 5) three to six times, then drop your knees to the ground and return to the kneeling position.

☺ *Easier.* If you find it uncomfortable or difficult to support the whole weight of your body with your back arched and your knees off the ground in steps 3 and 5, drop your pelvis to the ground and support only the weight of your head and trunk.

☺ *Harder*. From the arched position in step 5, as you exhale bend your elbows back, drop your shoulders and straighten your body so that you are looking at the floor with your body straight and parallel to the floor, supported on hands and feet. Hold your abdominal muscles tight for a few seconds after exhaling, and then breathe in as you return to the arch to continue with the rest of the exercise.

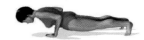

Forward bend and back arch

This arch uses passive flexion of the spine, but the thigh muscles, buttocks, erector spinae and shoulder muscles are used to hold the arch. It strengthens these muscles and mobilises the spinal joints.

1. Sit on the floor and slide your feet towards your buttocks until your thighs and lower legs are approximately at right angles. Take a deep breath in. As you breathe out, lean back with you head bent forward and place your hands on the floor behind you, fingers facing forward. Keep up the tension in your abdominal muscles as you pause for a few seconds.

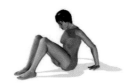

2. Without moving your hands or feet, as you inhale slowly push your pelvis forward and upward as high as you can, letting your head fall back as far as is comfortable. Pause for a few seconds. (If you wish you can exhale and inhale again in this position, keeping up the tension in your back and buttocks.)

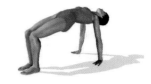

3. As you exhale, slowly lower yourself to the floor without moving your hands or feet and curl forward to the starting position. Keep up the tension in your abdominal muscles as you pause for a few seconds at the end of exhalation.

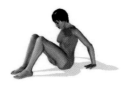

Repeat steps 2 and 3 three to six times.

Forward and backward bend sitting

This exercise mobilises the joints of your spine and strengthens both its extensors and its flexors. It also provides good strength training for your psoas muscles and the muscles of your thighs and abdominal wall.

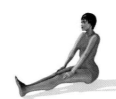

1. Sit on the floor with your legs straight out in front of you.

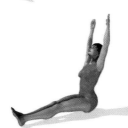

2. As you take a slow breath in, stretch your arms strongly above and behind your head and lean back, looking upward, until you feel your heels about to leave the floor. Hold this position for a few seconds at the end of the inhalation

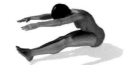

3. Exhaling, slowly lean forward, stretch your arms straight out in front of you as far as you can, looking downward. Hold your arm and abdominal muscles tight for a few seconds.

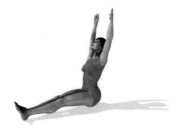

4. As you inhale, lean back and again stretch your arms strongly above and behind your head, looking upward until you feel your heels about to leave the floor. Hold this position for a few seconds at the end of the inhalation.

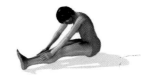

5. As you exhale, lean forward, drop you arms and grasp your legs below the knees, curl your spine, drop your head on to your chest and lower your chest towards your legs as far as you can comfortably. Hold your abdominal muscles tight for a few seconds at the end of exhalation.

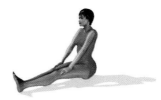

6. As you inhale, slowly uncurl, sliding you hands back along your legs and sit up tall.

7. Exhaling, slowly lie down, tilting your pelvis and curling your back as you let your vertebrae reach the floor one after the other: lower lumbar, upper lumbar and then thoracic. Keep looking forward and let your head down last.

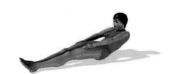

8. As you inhale, slowly raise your knees towards your chest.

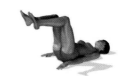

9. Still inhaling, straighten your legs until they are stretching straight up with the knee joints 'locked'. Hold that position for a few seconds at the end of inhalation.

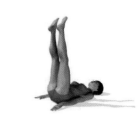

10. As you begin to exhale, lower your straightened legs slowly and smoothly to the floor.

11. Inhale slowly and draw your feet along the floor towards your buttocks, raising your knees, until you can feel the small of your back touching the floor. As you exhale reach forward, hook your fingers behind your thighs as high up as you can, raise you head and shoulders from the floor without pulling with your hands.

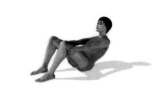

12. As you inhale, pull gently with your arms, straighten your legs and sit up slowly and smoothly.

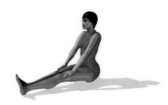

Do two to four complete repetitions, reaching further forward in step 5 each time until, if you can, you lock your fingers around your feet.

☺ *Harder.* Your neck and abdominal muscles can be given more strength training from the position after step 11. On inhalation, slowly lower your shoulders and then your head to the floor again. As you exhale hook your fingers behind your thighs, raise you head and shoulders from the floor without pulling with your hands. Raise and lower your head and shoulders four to six times, and then sit up to repeat the whole exercise.

Side bend standing

The *Side bend standing* mobilises the discs and the vertebral facet joints on each side. Strength training is given to the erector spinae muscles, the neck muscles, to the three layers of muscle that make up the sides of the abdominal wall and to the calf muscles. As usual, concentrate on what you are doing and feeling and don't let your mind wander.

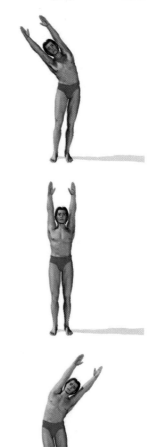

1. Stand with your feet a few inches apart. Take a slow breath in as you raise both arms strongly above your head and shift your weight to the balls of the feet without lifting your heels. Hold for a few seconds.

2. As you begin a slow exhalation, relax your shoulders, take your weight squarely on the soles of your feet and bend your arms, head and spine to the right, still looking forward. Firmly pull your head, neck, chest and trunk down to the right, taking all your weight on your right foot with the sole of your left foot resting lightly on the floor. Help the bend to the right by moving your pelvis slightly to the left. At the end of expiration, hold the tension for a few seconds.

3. Slowly straighten up as you begin a second slow inhalation, stretching your arms strongly above your head and shifting your weight to the balls of the feet without lifting your heels. Pause for a few seconds.

4. As you exhale, relax your shoulders, take your weight squarely on the soles of your feet and repeat the bend on the left side, moving your pelvis to the right. Firmly pull your head, neck, chest and trunk down to the left until all your weight is on your left foot with your right foot resting lightly on the floor.

Repeat three to six times on each side.

&. *Disabled.* The bends can be done seated.

Side pull standing

This works on the same spinal joints as the *Side bend standing* but mobilises them a little further by fixing the pelvis.

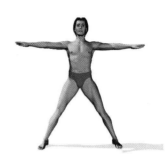

1. Stand with your feet two or three feet apart, so that you can feel the muscles on the inner sides of your thighs being gently stretched As you begin a slow breath in, slowly raise your arms sideways until they are horizontal and extend them strongly sideways as far as you can. Hold briefly.

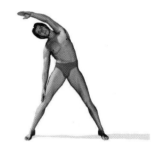

2. As you begin to exhale, pull your head, neck and trunk firmly down to the right still looking forward, reach firmly downward with your right arm until your hand is near or below your right knee, and slowly swing your left arm over your head to reach as far to the right as is comfortable. Make sure you shoulders stay in line with your feet and you do not lean forward. Hold the tension for a few seconds at the end of expiration.

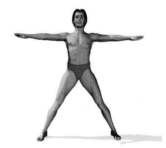

3. As you breathe in, straighten up with your arms horizontal, reaching out strongly sideways. Pause briefly at the end of inspiration.

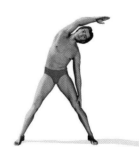

4. Repeat the stretch on the other side, pulling your head, neck and trunk firmly down to the left, again making sure that you do not lean forward.

Do three to six repetitions of the complete exercise.

&. *Disabled.* The bends can be done seated.

Body roll standing

The body roll takes your spine through a sequence of bends like those of the stick used by a Chinese plate juggler. The spinal facet joints and the discs are mobilised as the spine flexes, bends sideways, extends and bends to the other side. All the muscles that bend the spine are used.

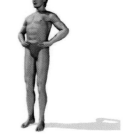

1. Stand with your feet a few inches apart and place your hands on your hips. Take a slow breath in.

2. As you begin to breathe out, slowly curl your spine forward until you are looking at the floor. Hold the tension in your abdominal muscles for a few seconds at the end of exhalation.

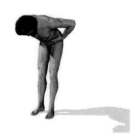

3. Roll your head and spine to the right as you start a second slow inhalation, looking forward. Firmly pull your head, neck, chest and trunk down to the right until all your weight is being taken on your right foot and your left foot has almost no pressure on the floor. Help the bend to the right by gently pressing on your right hip with your right hand. At the end of inspiration, hold the tension for a few seconds.

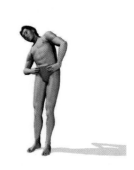

4. Exhale slowly, roll your spine gently backward as you pull your head back and look upward. Help the backward curve by gently pushing your pelvis forward with both hands. Hold the tension briefly.

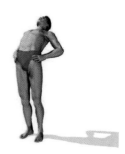

5. As you inhale, roll your head and spine slowly around to the left. Again look forward as you firmly pull your head, neck, chest and trunk down to the left until all your weight is being taken on your left foot and your right foot has almost no pressure on the floor. Help the bend to the left by gently pressing on your left hip with your left hand.

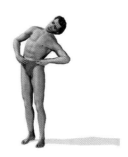

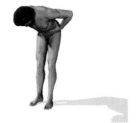

6. During slow exhalation, roll forward to the starting position. Hold the tension in your abdominal muscles for a few seconds at the end of exhalation.

Do two to four rolls to the right, and then repeat two or three times rolling the other way.

☺ *Harder.* Instead of keeping your hands on your hips, raise both arms strongly above your head as you take the first slow inhalation. Keep them extended as they follow the rolling motion of your body forwards, sideways, backwards, sideways and forwards again. This provides strength training for the shoulder muscles and, because of the weight of your arms, additional resistance for the spinal muscles.

♿ *Disabled.* Similar movements over a smaller range can be carried out while seated.

Half sideways bend and twist sitting

The bending of the spine in this exercise is half way between front to back and side to side. It provides strength training for your thigh and shoulder muscles as well as exercising your spinal flexors and extensors.

1. Sit on the floor with your legs stretched out sideways as far apart as is comfortable and take a slow breath in.

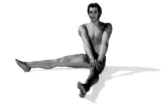

2. As you exhale, slowly lean forward towards your left foot, stretch your arms out in front of you as far as you can and look downward. Hold your arm and abdominal muscles tight for a few seconds.

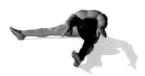

3. As you inhale lean back and to the right in line with your left leg, look upward and stretch your arms strongly above and behind your head until you feel all your weight on your right buttock and your left heel is just about to leave the floor. Hold this position for a few seconds at the end of the inhalation.

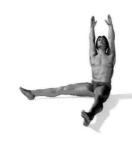

4. As you exhale, slowly swing your arms down, curl your spine and grasp your left leg somewhere below the knee. Pull your head in to your chest and lower your chest towards your thigh as far as you can comfortably, trying to touch your knee with your forehead. Hold your abdominal muscles tight for a few seconds at the end of exhalation.

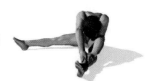

5. As you inhale, slowly uncurl, sliding you hands back along your left leg. Then turn to the right so that you are looking at your right foot. Hold this position for a few seconds at the end of the inhalation.

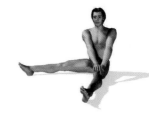

6. Exhaling, slowly lean forward towards your right foot, stretch your arms out in front of you as far as you can and look downward.

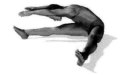

7. As you inhale, lean back and to the left in line with your right leg, look up and stretch your arms strongly above and behind your head until you feel all your weight on your left buttock and your right heel is about to leave the floor. Hold this position for a few seconds at the end of the inhalation.

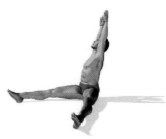

8. As you exhale, lean forward and grasp your right leg as you did on the other side. Pull your head in to your chest and lower your chest towards your thigh as far as you can comfortably, trying to touch your knee with your forehead. Hold your abdominal muscles tight for a few seconds at the end of exhalation.

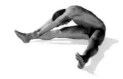

Do two to four complete repetitions, reaching further forward each time until, if you can, you lock your fingers around your feet.

☺ *Harder.* Place the sole of your right foot against your the inner side of your thigh in your left groin before starting. Do two to four repetitions on that side, then place your left foot in your right groin and repeat on the other side.

Side raise lying

This exercise exerts considerable pressure on your hip, so it is important to lie on something like a pillow or a folded blanket that is thick enough to provide adequate padding. It strengthens your thigh and buttock muscles and the muscle layers of the side walls of your abdomen, and mobilises the discs and vertebral facet joints in your lumbar region.

1. Lie on your left side with your right leg resting on your left leg and your head supported by your left hand. Place your right hand flat on the floor six to nine inches in front of your chest with the fingers pointing away from your feet. Take a slow breath in and pause.

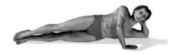

2. As you breathe out, push down firmly on the floor with your right hand and slowly raise both legs sideways as high as is comfortable, keeping in position as you pause at the end of exhalation and take a slow breath in.

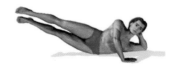

3. As you breathe out, slowly lower both legs to the floor again.

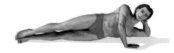

4. Relax as you take a slow breath in, pause, and then repeat from step 2.

Do three to six bends on the left side and then an equal number on the right.

☺ *Easier.* Raise only the upper leg.

Chapter 7: Twists

Twist standing

Twisting is often the first of the spinal movements to lose flexibility. The spine is rotated about its length, mobilising the facet joints and discs. The movements strengthen the neck, prevertebral, erector spinae, transverse abdominal and psoas muscles. The deltoid muscles at the top of the shoulders are also strengthened because they are in action throughout. Try to concentrate on what you are doing and feeling and don't let your mind wander.

1. Stand with your feet a few inches apart. As you begin a slow inhalation, raise your arms straight in front of you and hold your right thumb with your left hand. Extend your arms firmly forward so that your chest muscles stand out, take your weight on the balls of your feet and pause for a few seconds.

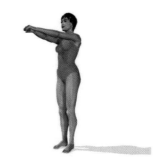

2. As you begin a slow exhalation, relax the shoulder tension and take your weight squarely on your feet. Turn your pelvis to the right, then your chest, shoulders and arms, then your head and neck and finally your eyes, all in one smooth movement. Hold the extreme position firmly for a few seconds at the end of exhalation.

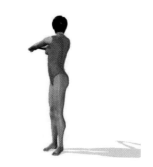

3. As you begin the next slow inhalation, slowly rotate around to the front, first moving the pelvis, then the chest, shoulders and arms, then the head, neck and eyes. Again extend your arms firmly forward, take your weight on the balls of your feet and pause for a few seconds.

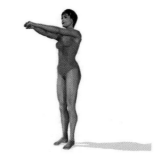

4. Hold your left thumb with your right hand as you begin to exhale slowly and twist to the left side, first your pelvis, then your chest, shoulders and arms, then your head and neck and finally your eyes. Hold the extreme position firmly for a few seconds at the end of exhalation.

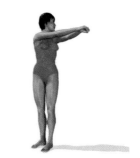

5. As you begin the next slow inhalation, slowly rotate around to the front, again first moving the pelvis, then the chest, shoulders and arms, then the head, neck and eyes. Extend your arms firmly forward and take your weight on the balls of your feet as before.

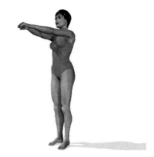

Repeat three to six times on each side.

☺ *Harder.* Rise on your toes as you twist. Lower your feet as you turn to the front.

♿ *Disabled.* Similar movements can be carried out over a slightly smaller range while seated.

Twist sitting

This exercise also rotates your spine around its length, strengthening your neck, prevertebral, erector spinae, and transverse abdominal muscles and mobilising the facet joints and discs. The position of your legs prevents the pelvis from turning, so the muscles can twist your spine more strongly than in the *Twist standing*.

1. Place the sole of your right foot against the inner side of your thigh in your left groin. Then lift your left foot and place it on the floor to the right of your right knee. Make sure you are sitting up straight as you take a slow breath in and pause.

2. As you exhale, slowly turn to the left, reaching over your left knee with your right hand to hold your right knee, with your elbow against your left thigh. Twist first your chest and shoulders, then your head, then your eyes. Sit tall with no weight on your left hand. Turn as far as is comfortable, hold your abdominal muscles tight and pause. (If you wish, you can hold this position while taking a slow breath in and out, turning a little further as you exhale if you are able to do so comfortably.)

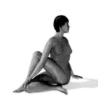

43

3. As you breathe in, slowly return to the starting position, moving first your chest, then you head and then your eyes.

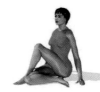

Repeat the twist three to six times to the left and then change the position of your legs and repeat an equal number of times to the right.

☺ *Easier.* If you find the leg position difficult, sit with both legs straight out in front of you, cross you left leg over your right leg and reach over it to hold your right knee with your right hand.

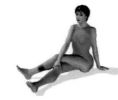

Twist lying

This twist concentrates on the facet joints of the lower part of your spine and on your hip joints. It strengthens the erector spinae, transverse abdominal and psoas muscles, and also the muscles of your thighs.

1. Lie on your back with your legs straight and your arms on the floor palms down at about 45 degrees to your body.

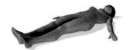

2. As you begin a slow breath in, keep your right leg straight and in contact with the floor and slowly raise you left thigh with the knee bent.

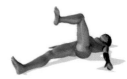

3. Still inhaling, extend your leg until it is stretching straight up with the knee joint 'locked'. Hold the extended position for a few seconds after completing the inhalation.

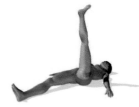

4. As you begin to breathe out, slowly twist your pelvis to the right and lower your left leg towards the floor on the left in line with your hips, making sure that both of your shoulders remain in contact with the floor. Hold this position for a few seconds after exhalation is complete. (If you wish you can hold this position for a further slow breath. As you exhale, gently press on the floor with your left hand to twist a little further to the right.)

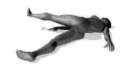

5. As you begin to inhale, slowly twist your pelvis back so that it is flat on the floor again as you raise your left leg to the vertical position. Hold the extended position briefly after completing inhalation.

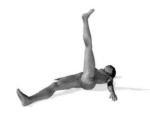

6. As you exhale, slowly lower your extended left leg to the floor.

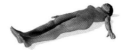

Do three to six repetitions alternately on each side. When you have become sufficiently supple to touch the floor with the toes of your extended leg in line with your hips, aim to touch the floor as near to your head as you can.

☺ *Easier.* Instead of extending your leg, you can draw both your knees towards your chest and then twist your pelvis with your knees bent.

☺ *Harder.* Raise both legs at the same time, keeping them extended together with the knees 'locked' as you twist your pelvis.

Forward bend and twist standing

The spinal facet joints are mobilised by rotation of your spine while it is flexed. It strengthens your shoulder, back and neck muscles as well as those of your spine.

1. Stand facing forward with your feet two or three feet apart, so that you can feel the muscles on the inner sides of your thighs being gently stretched. Take a slow breath in as you raise your arms horizontally in line with your legs and extend them strongly sideways as far as you can.

2. As you exhale, slowly bend forward and hold your right ankle or foot with your left hand. As you twist, raise your right arm above your head and turn your head to the right as you try to look at the hand. Hold this position for a few seconds at the end of exhalation. (If you wish, hold this position for a further slow breath. As you exhale, gently pull with your left hand to twist a little further to the right.)

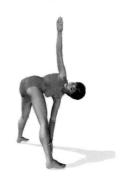

3. As you inhale, slowly straighten up so that you are again standing erect looking forward with your arms extended strongly sideways.

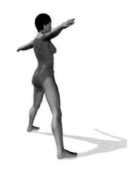

4. As you exhale repeat the twist from step 2 on the left side.

Do three to six repetitions on each side.

☺ *Easier.* If you cannot reach low down your right leg with your left hand or *vice versa*, try the same exercise with your feet closer together. Instead of stretching the other arm upward, you can rest your hand on the back of your hip on the same side.

☺ *Harder.* When you become sufficiently flexible, instead of holding the opposite ankle or foot, place your hand flat on the floor outside the opposite foot.

Sideways bend and twist standing

The spinal facet joints are further mobilised by rotation of your spine while it is bent sideways. The muscles of your shoulders, back and neck as well as those of your spine are strengthened.

1. Stand facing forward with your feet two or three feet apart, so that you can feel the muscles on the inner sides of your thighs being gently stretched. Turn your left foot on the heel until it is pointing to the left. Lift your right heel and swivel it backward on the ball of the foot until it is at 45 degrees as shown in the picture. Take a slow breath in as you raise your arms horizontally in line with your legs and extend them strongly sideways as far as you can.

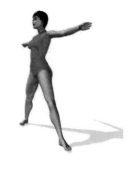

2. As you breathe out, slowly bend down to the left, reach as far as you can with your left hand and grasp the front of your leg or ankle. Do not let your pelvis move back so that you bend forward at the hip. At the same time raise your right arm above your head and turn your head to the right as you try to look at the hand. Pause briefly. (If you wish, hold this position for a further slow breath. As you exhale gently push backward with your left hand and let your right arm 'fall' backward to twist a little further.)

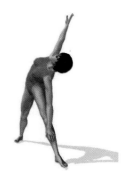

3. As you inhale, slowly straighten up and twist to the left so that you are again standing erect looking forward with your arms extended strongly sideways.

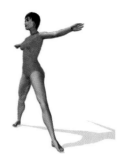

Do three to six repetitions to the left, change the position of your feet and do an equal number to the right.

☺ *Harder.* As you become more flexible, you may find that you can lower the raised arm behind your back, reach forward with your hand and grasp the top of the opposite thigh.

Chapter 8: Straight spine exercises

Hand clasp

This exercise increases the flexibility of your shoulder joints. It strengthens your forearm, upper arm, shoulder and upper back muscles. It is particularly important to use the easier variation if you begin to experience any discomfort at all. As usual, breathe slowly, concentrate on what you are doing and feeling, and don't let your mind wander.

1. Stand with your feet a few inches apart.

2. Swing your left hand behind you as high up as you can reach so that the back of your hand is against your spine and the palm is facing backward.

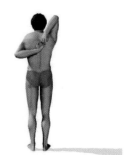

3. As you begin a slow breath in, raise your right hand behind your head, palm facing forward and slide it down your spine so that you can link fingers with your left hand. Pull gently upward and to the right with your right arm. Try to make sure that your right elbow is pointing sideways, but don't worry if you can't do this at first. Keep your head up straight, chin tucked in, looking forward.

4. As you breathe out, gently pull your linked hands downward and to the left with your left arm.

5. As you breathe in, release your fingers, swing your right hand behind you as far up as you can reach and repeat on the other side.

Repeat three to six times.

☺   *Easier.* If your shoulders are stiff and you find you cannot link your hands behind you, or if you experience any discomfort, hold a scarf, tie or something similar in the upper hand and grasp it with the lower hand as you do the pulls.

♿   *Disabled.* This exercise can be done seated.

Squat

This exercise strengthens your calf muscles and those in the front of your lower legs, the hamstrings and the muscles in the front of your thighs, the psoas muscles, the muscles of your buttocks and the erector spinae. It also provides some work for your arms and shoulders. It helps to improve your balance.

1. Stand with your feet a few inches apart and take a slow breath in.

2. As you begin a slow breath out, stretch your arms out firmly downward and forward so that the muscles in the front of your chest (the pectorals) stand out, and lean forward as you slowly squat down to the point where your heels are just about to leave the ground. Pause with your abdominal muscles held tight.

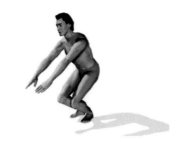

3. Slowly breathe in as you rise to a standing position again.

Repeat three to six times.

☺   *Easier.* Extend your arms in front of you and grasp the back or seat of a chair as you squat. If you have hip or knee problems, make sure you take the squat only as far as is comfortable.

☺ *Harder.* During the first slow breath in, raise your arms sideways and press the palms of your hands together immediately above your head, fingers pointing upward and elbows pointing sideways. As you breathe out, keep up the hand pressure as you slowly drop to a complete squat, sitting on your heels with your knees fully flexed. Pause with your abdominal muscles held tight. Slowly rise to the standing position as you breathe in.

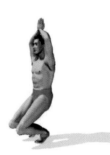

🛋 *Pregnancy.* Start with your feet 12 to 18 inches apart, knees pointing outwards at about 45 degrees, and hold on to a chair if you wish. This produces only gentle abdominal pressure. Practising squatting regularly during pregnancy is said to make for an easier birth.

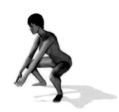

Forward arm and leg pull

This balancing posture helps to mobilise your hip, knee and ankle joints. It strengthens the muscles that raise your shoulders, the biceps muscles and the muscles that flex your forearms. Because it involves standing on one leg it also strengthens your front and side thigh muscles and the muscles of your bottom and back.

1. As you take a slow breath in, raise your right foot and rest it on your left knee, lean forward and grasp your right knee with your right hand and your right foot with your left hand, palm facing forward.

2. As you breathe out, slowly pull your knee towards your chest and pull your foot upward, keeping it in the midline. Do not pull harder or further than is comfortable.

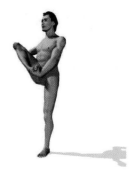

3. Take a slow breath in as you hold this position, keeping up the tension.

4. As you exhale, slowly return your foot to the floor.

Repeat on the other side and do three to six complete repetitions.

△ *Warning.* Until you are certain of your balance it is wise to start with your back to a wall with your heels two or three inches from it, preferably in a corner, so that you can lean backward if you feel unsteady. Alternatively, the posture can be done sitting on the front edge of a chair or stool or lying on one's back.

Backward arm and leg pull

Like the *Forward arm and leg pull* this balancing posture helps to mobilise your hip, knee and ankle joints. It also strengthens your shoulder and arm muscles, and the muscles involved in standing on one leg.

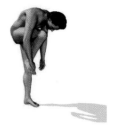

1. As you take a slow breath in, raise you right knee, lean forward and grasp the front of your ankle.

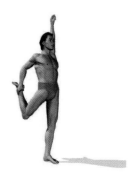

2. As you exhale, pull you right foot backward and upward as far as is comfortable. At the same time, raise your left arm strongly above your head.

3. Take a slow breath in as you hold this position with your back straight, keeping up the muscle tension.

4. As you exhale, slowly return your foot to the floor and drop your arm to your side.

Repeat on the other side and do three to six complete repetitions.

△ *Warning.* Until you are certain of your balance it is wise to start standing sideways to a wall with you feet six or eight inches away so that you can rest your raised arm on it.

☺ *Harder.* This extension changes the straight spine posture into a backward bend, mobilising the spinal joints. As you exhale in step 2, lean forward, keeping your head upright, and pull your foot up until your thigh is parallel with the floor.

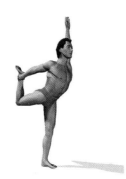

All fours

This strenuous exercise strengthens the muscles of your arms and shoulders, back and legs.

1. Kneel on the floor with your knees a couple of inches apart and sit on your heels.

2. Take a slow breath in as you place your hands flat on the floor as close to you knees as you can, with the fingers pointing towards each other and your elbows straight. Tuck your toes under.

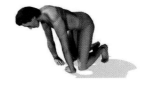

3. As you breathe out, straighten your legs, rise on your toes and lean as far forward as you can, looking at your hands. Hold your abdominal muscles tight as you pause.

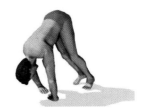

4. As you breathe in, move your body backward as far as you can, if possible with the soles of your feet flat on the floor. Relax your neck and look towards your feet. Hold this position for a few seconds at the end of the breath.

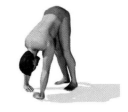

5. As you begin to take the next slow breath out, keep your legs straight and move your body as far forward as you can again. Hold this position for a few seconds at the end of the breath.

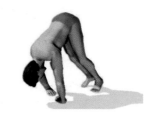

6. As you breathe in, slowly bend your knees, lower your body and return to the starting position.

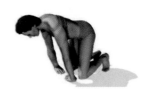

Repeat three to six times.

SECTION 3: CHOOSING HOW TO EXERCISE

Chapter 9: Preparing for a *Slow Yoga* session

You would be wise to consult your doctor before starting any program of flexibility exercises, including *Slow Yoga*

- If you are under medical care
- If you have painful joints
- If you have persistent pains in the back, neck, shoulder, arm, wrist, buttock, thigh or calf
- If you have weakness, tingling or numbness anywhere.

When and where ?

It is best not to practise *Slow Yoga* immediately after waking up. During sleep, fluid moves out of the circulation into the tissues, tending to make joints stiffer and muscles less flexible first thing in the morning. Yoga should never be practised on a full stomach, so the best time is after being up and about for a while but before breakfast. If you like, have a glass of water, fruit juice or milk, or a cup of tea or coffee, and then take a warm bath or shower. The warmth and towelling dry will loosen your muscles and joints.

An alternative times for a session are before your midday or evening meal. In the evening try winding down from the stresses of the day by practising a breathing exercise such as the *Slow breath lying* (p 12) for a few minutes before starting. This will help to 'halt the whirlings of the mind' and relieve muscular tension.

If you smoke, you would be very wise to give up for the sake of your general health. In any event, you should refrain from smoking for at least two hours before exercise; smoking causes a substantial reduction in the blood supply to the discs and spinal facet joints which takes up to two hours to return to normal.

Slow Yoga can be practised anywhere, indoors or outdoors – but it should be a quiet place with nothing to distract the mind from being receptive to the sensations arising from the exercises. Your own bedroom or sitting room may be the best place.

Clothing and equipment

The exercises should always be done with bare feet because you will need to stand on your toes or bend them. Clothing, if any, should be light and not restricting. Trousers should have an elastic waistband rather than a belt. You will need something comfortable to lie on; even a carpeted floor does not provide enough padding. A thick beach towel folded lengthways is ideal. If possible, practise in front of a full-length mirror in the early stages so that you can check your positions.

Little equipment is used for *Slow Yoga*, and none is essential. A small pillow or a cushion is useful to support the head in the *Slow breath lying* (p 12), to sit on cross-legged for *Alternate nostril breathing* (p 11), to pad the hip in *Side raise lying* (p 41) and, if necessary, to support the shoulders in the *Shoulder stand* (p 9). Holding a scarf or tie between the hands is the easiest way to start doing the *Hand clasp* (p 48).

How long and how often?

Research has shown that muscles develop maximum strength with about five repetitions of reasonably strong five to ten second contractions repeated on five or more days a week. *Slow Yoga* strength training is based on this research finding. In each resistance exercise the five to ten second contractions are repeated up to six times, and a program of exercises is chosen so as to cover a wide range of muscles. Movements are synchronised with very slow breathing. It takes 20-40 minutes for you to complete the kind of example programs given on pages 58 to 63. A session could be split into two 10-20 minute sessions if that were more convenient, although each of them would benefit from some kind of warm-up. Even one ten-minute session is better than nothing. *Slow Yoga* is enjoyable, and 20 minutes or so five days a week is a small commitment for all the benefits that follow.

Attending a class with an instructor once a week is not 'doing Yoga'. Strength and flexibility start being lost if you have more than two or three days between sessions. For this reason, if you do attend a class you should supplement it with daily home practice. Make sure that what is being taught is the kind of thing you want to learn. There are several schools of Yoga (p 75). Some of them, for example *Astanga Yoga* or *Power Yoga*, are suitable for young fit people. However, unlike *Slow Yoga*, you would not be able to carry them on into your seventies, eighties and nineties. Individual attention from the instructor is essential, and you are not likely to get that if there are more than, say, six in a class. The dangers of class Yoga are that the other pupils can easily distract you, and that there is a tendency for sessions to become competitive. If you have been taught some Yoga postures you enjoy, you can adapt them to include strength training by incorporating the principles of *Slow Yoga* (p 20).

Gain without pain

During *Slow Yoga* you need an active relaxed body and a passive, alert and receptive mind. It is important to concentrate on what you are doing and on the sensations you experience because they can warn you when you are overdoing things. When you start using slow controlled breathing you need to look out for the warning symptoms of over-breathing (p 5) and slow your breathing rate down. The earliest symptoms are a light-headed feeling and 'pins and needles' around the mouth and in the fingers. You should always breathe through your nose and not your mouth. You may hear creaking, grating, crunching or popping noises from your joints when you start exercising. You can safely ignore them unless they are painful.

You will experience the pleasant sensations of muscles contracting strongly and of muscles, ligaments and joints stretching. Concentrate on letting go of the tension in muscles that are being stretched so that you can pull a little further each time, but never carry stretching to the point where it produces discomfort. Pain produces a reflex contraction of muscle to protect the injured part, and continuing to stretch may cause soft tissue injury. Move slowly so that muscles that are lengthening are not under tension. Moving rapidly, for example bouncing down to touch your toes, lets the momentum of the movement pull hard on muscles that have not relaxed. It can produce severe pain due the tearing of muscle fibres, ligaments or even tendons. You may not notice a minor degree of injury during the session, but afterwards there is likely to be persistent localised pain, tenderness and muscle spasm that can take as long as six weeks to recover. Be particularly careful if you exercise after you have taken an analgesic such as paracetamol or ibuprofen for aches and pains because you may not experience the sensations that warn of damage.

After a session you will feel the warm pleasant glow of muscles that have been exercised vigorously. An unpleasant sensation of general muscle soreness usually means you have pushed yourself too hard or carried out too many repetitions of the same exercise.

If you concentrate on what you are doing and pay attention to what you feel, you will gain without pain.

Chapter 10: Planning Slow Yoga programs

You can devise daily programs to use at home by choosing one, two or three exercises from each of the five spinal movement groups listed in the Table. It is best to choose them so that they flow easily from one to the other using a sequence like standing, on hands and knees, sitting and then lying, or *vice versa*. If you were away from home without a mat you could choose a sequence entirely from the standing exercises.

It is a good idea to begin with a slow breathing exercise. This will reinforce the importance of slow breathing synchronised with slow movement. It will also let you concentrate on achieving the slowest breathing pace that you can maintain, so you can carry that slow pace forward into the rest of the session. A second slow breathing exercise at the end is useful to allow you to wind down and relax.

Some suggestions for *Slow Yoga* programs follow the Table. Both the programs and the exercises themselves can be modified: anything that feels right is right. Remember that you can adapt Yoga postures you already know and enjoy to incorporate the strength training principles of *Slow Yoga* (p 20). The first program uses movements that those new to Yoga can adapt to most readily. It is probably best not to move on to the other programs until you have completely mastered the first. When you do move on, start with the easier versions of the programs (☺) for the first week or two. One way of making sure that you experience a full range of exercises and train most of your muscles and joints is to use the five programs in sequence, perhaps one on each of the five weekdays. When you feel like a challenge, you might think about introducing some of the harder variations (☻).

☞ *Pregnancy.* The exercises in the sixth set are designed for the later months of pregnancy They accommodate the baby during bending and none of them exerts pressure on the abdomen. The *Squat* modified for pregnancy (p 49) stretches the inner side of the thighs and opens up the pelvis. Practising squatting regularly during pregnancy is said to make for an easier birth. The *Forward and backward bend on hands and knees* (p 30) strengthens the abdominal and spinal muscles and the muscles that form the floor of the pelvis. You could include both in the program every day. It is useful to continue to practise the *Forward and backward bend on hands and knees* several times a day for a few weeks after delivery of the baby to help the muscles of the abdominal wall and pelvic floor return to normal.

♿ *Disabled.* There are a number of exercises that do not involve the legs: *Slow alternate nostril breathing* (p 11) , *Slow breath lying* (p 12), *Forward and backward bend sitting* (omitting the leg movements, p 33), *Twist sitting* (p 43) and *Hand clasp* (p 48). The arm and spine movements of several exercises can be carried out sitting on a chair or a stool: *Slow breath and stretch* (p 8), *Back arch standing* (p 22), *Forward and backward bend standing* (p 28), *Side bend* (p 36), *Side pull* (p 37) and *Body roll standing* (p 38). The first four of the 'office' exercises described later in Chapter 12 (p 69) are also suitable.

MAIN *SLOW YOGA* EXERCISES

Slow breathing (p 6)	Slow breath standing	Slow breath and stretch	Shoulder stand (slow breath upside-down)	Slow alternate nostril breathing	Slow breath lying
Backward bends (p 22)	Back arch standing	Back arch lying	Chest and neck arch prone	Leg and lumbar arch prone	Back arch prone
Forward and backward bends (p 28)	Forward and backward bend standing	Forward and backward bend on hands and knees	Forward and backward bend on hands and feet	Forward bend and back arch	Forward and backward bend sitting
Sideways bends (p 36)	Side bend standing	Side pull standing	Body roll standing	Half sideways bend and twist sitting	Side raise lying
Twists (p 42)	Twist standing	Twist sitting	Twist lying	Forward bend and twist standing	Sideways bend and twist standing
Straight spine exercises (p 48)	Hand clasp	Squat	Forward arm and leg pull	Backward arm and leg pull	All fours

Program 1

1. Slow breath standing, 3-8 slow breaths (p 6)

2. Forward and backward bend standing, 2-4 times (p 28)

3. Side bend standing, 3-6 times on each side (p 36)

4. Twist standing, 3-6 times on each side (p 42)

5. Squat, 3-6 times (p 48)

6. Back arch lying, 3-6 times (p 23)

7. Slow alternate nostril breathing, 5-10 slow breaths (p 11)

Program 2

1. Slow breath and stretch, 3-8 slow breaths (p 8)

2. Side pull standing, 3-6 times on each side (p 37)

3. Back arch standing, 3-6 times each way (p 22)

4. Hand clasp, 3-6 times on each side (p 48)

5. Forward & backward bend on hands & knees, 3-6 times (p 30)

6. Twist sitting, 3-6 times each way (p 43)

7. Shoulder stand, 5-10 slow breaths (p 9)

or Slow alternate nostril breathing, 5-10 slow breaths (p 11)

Program 3

1. Slow breath and stretch, 3-8 slow breaths (p 8)

2. Body roll standing, 2-4 times each way (p 38)

3. Forward arm and leg pull, 3-6 times on each side (p 49)

4. Forward & backward bend on hands & feet, 3-6 times (p 30)

5. Twist lying, 3-6 times each way (p 44)

6. Chest and neck arch prone, 3-6 times (p 24)

7. Shoulder stand, 5-10 slow breaths (p 9)

or Slow alternate nostril breathing, 5-10 slow breaths (p 11)

Program 4

1. Slow breath and stretch, 5-10 slow breaths (p 8)

2. Forward bend and twist standing, 3-6 times on each side (p 45)

3. Backward arm and leg pull, 3-6 times on each side (p 50)

4. Forward and backward bend sitting, 2-4 times (p 33)

5. Leg & lumbar arch prone, 3-6 times (p 25)

6. Side raise lying, 3-6 times (p 41)

7. Shoulder stand, 5-10 slow breaths (p 9)

or Slow alternate nostril breathing, 5-10 slow breaths (p 11)

Program 5

1. Slow breath and stretch, 5-10 slow breaths (p 8)

2. Sideways bend and twist standing, 3-6 times on each side (p 46)

3. Half sideways bend & twist sitting, 2-4 times on each side (p 39)

4. Forward bend and back arch, 3-6 times (p 32)

5. Back arch prone, 3-6 times (p 26)

6. All fours, 3-6 times (p 51)

7. Shoulder stand, 5-10 slow breaths (p 9)

or Slow alternate nostril breathing, 5-10 slow breaths (p 11)

Program 6 (pregnancy)

After the third month all exercises should be done gently because pregnancy makes your ligaments and joint capsules more flexible and more easily stretched.

1. Slow breath lying in pregnancy, 5-10 slow breaths (p 13)

2. Twist sitting, easier version, 3-6 times (p 43)

3. Forward & backward bend on hands and knees, 3-6 times (p 30)

4. Forward & backward bend standing in pregnancy, 3-4 times (p 28)

5. Side pull standing, 3-6 times (p 37)

6. Squat in pregnancy, 3-6 times (p 49)

7. Slow alternate nostril breathing, 5-10 slow breaths (p 11)

Bad Yoga

△ *Warning.* There are some conventional Yoga postures that are of little value, are unwise and may be dangerous.

There seems to be little point in Westerners spending time and effort in attempting to achieve the full cross-legged *Lotus* posture. BKS Iyengar, a famous Indian teacher of Yoga, wrote that people who are not used to sitting on the floor will feel excruciating pain around the knees at first that will subside with perseverance. If it hurts, why persevere? During exercises like *Slow alternate nostril breathing* (p 11) there is no reason why you should not sit on the floor in a comfortable cross-legged position (on a cushion if you prefer) or on a stool or a chair.

The *Headstand* is a potentially dangerous posture that puts a great deal of pressure on the cervical (neck) vertebrae and discs. It can lead to pain in the neck, shoulders and arm and a chronically stiff neck. It is a common cause of falls even when practised in the corner of a room with potential support from the walls. It has no advantage over the much safer *Shoulder stand* (p 9).

Any posture that can lead to the weight of the body bending the neck backward should be avoided. For example, there is a harder version of the *Back arch lying* (p 23) called the *Wheel* that is not included in this book. After raising the pelvis and making an arch, the hands reach upward and backward and are placed on the ground near the shoulders, fingers pointing towards the feet. The shoulders are then raised off the ground by pushing with the hands and feet, the top of the head contacts the floor and the neck is extended. A final push with the arms completes a full arch supported on the hands and feet. There are a number of case reports in the medical literature of vertebral artery thrombosis following hyperextension of the neck in this way resulting in permanent neurological damage. The *Forward bend and back arch* (p 32) achieves the same posture without the risk of body weight hyperextending the neck. Another posture not included in this book, the *Fish*, also hyperextends the neck and should be avoided for the same reason. The *Chest and neck arch prone* (p 24) exercises the same groups of muscles without risk.

Some articles in the medical literature have ascribed ill effects to Yoga unfairly. For example, a young woman died from air embolism after practising what the author called 'Yoga breathing exercises' – but these involved mouth-to-mouth breathing with a boy friend in a dance hall filled with marijuana smoke. Yoga was also blamed in three separate case reports for foot-drop: the first in a male professor who fell asleep for three hours in the lotus position; the second in a young woman who meditated in the lotus position for hours; and the third in a young man who knelt sitting on his heels for six hours while chanting for world peace. All three recovered spontaneously. These reports show how important it is to remain alert and concentrate on what you are doing and feeling when practising Yoga, even when meditating (p 93).

Chapter 11: Exercises while shaving or making up

Most of us spend some time each day looking at our faces in a mirror, either shaving or making up. The activity has usually been repeated so often that it has become automatic and requires little thought. These exercises have been designed to strengthen the muscles of your abdominal wall, back, buttocks and thighs and to mobilise the facet joints of the lower end of your spine without interfering with the semi-automatic activity that is going on at the same time. Try to concentrate on your breathing and hip movements, and on making sure your chest, shoulders and feet do not move rather than on what you see in the mirror.

The exercises can also be used several times a day in the early stages after an attack of incapacitating low back pain to help with recovery. The movements should be pushed to the edge of discomfort but not beyond.

Pelvic tilt

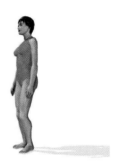

1. Standing erect, bend you knees so that your body is lowered two or three inches.

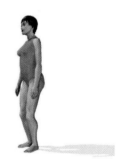

2. As you take a slow breath in, tilt your pelvis back so that the hollow of your back is increased and you can feel the muscles on each side of your spine contracting hard. Pause for two or three seconds in full inspiration.

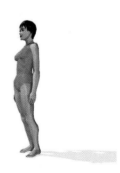

3. As you slowly exhale, tilt the pelvis forward and upward, contracting the buttocks and the muscles of the floor of the pelvis – the muscle groups that are used to prevent accidents when one has diarrhoea or a full bladder and that contract during orgasm. Make sure your head and shoulders do not move. Keep up the tension as you pause for a few seconds at the end of expiration.

Repeat the movements with each slow breath as often as you like.

Pelvic twist

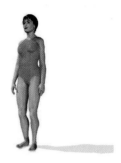

1. Stand erect with the knees very slightly bent, not locked, and take your weight on the balls of your feet, keeping your heels in contact with the floor. Breathe in slowly and pause for a few seconds.

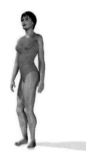

2. As you exhale, take your weight squarely on your feet and twist your pelvis slowly and firmly to the right, making sure that your feet and shoulders do not move. Keep the muscles on the right side of your abdomen and spine firm as you pause.

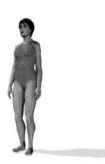

3. Breathe in slowly as you twist back to the starting position, again taking your weight on the balls of your feet and keeping your heels in contact with the floor. Pause for a few seconds

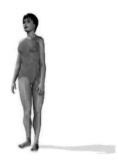

4. Repeat the twist on the other side.

Repeat the movements on each side as often as you like.

Pelvic roll

1. Standing erect, bend you knees so that your body is lowered two or three inches.

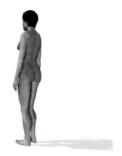

2. As you take a slow breath in, tilt your pelvis back so that the hollow of your back is increased in the same way as you did in the *Pelvic tilt*. Pause for two or three seconds in full inspiration.

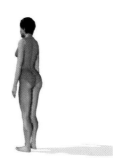

3. As you breathe out, swing your pelvis to the right by bending your left knee and straightening your right leg.

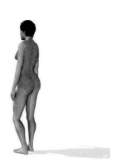

4. While you are still exhaling, straighten both legs, tilt your pelvis forward and upward in the same way as you did in the *Pelvis tilt*, making sure your head and shoulders do not move. Hold your abdominal muscles tight at the end of expiration.

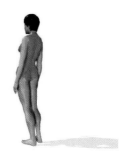

5. As you breathe in, swing your pelvis to the left by bending you right knee and straightening your left.

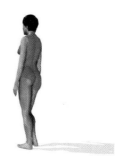

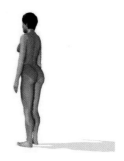

6. While you are still inhaling, tilt your pelvis back to the position in step 2 with your knees slightly bent. Hold your lower back muscles tight as you pause.

Either continue with one or two rolls in the same direction and then a similar number the other way, or reverse direction every time you reach the position in steps 2 and 6.

Chapter 12: Exercises in the office and travelling

The human body is designed for movement. When it remains still for long periods the muscles and joints become stiff. If a poor sitting or standing posture compounds the immobility, the spinal nerve windows are narrowed and cause discomfort or pain.

Many of us have jobs that require us to remain still, for example sitting at a desk operating office equipment, while others have to sit still while travelling. It is natural to feel the need to move around when there is a chance. If you have space you can use any of the *Slow Yoga* exercises that were given earlier in the book. The exercises below suggest some of the movements that that will help to relieve the aches, pains and stiffness of relative immobility where space is restricted. The exercises can all be done seated.

Neck roll

1. Sit tall and upright with your shoulders and arms relaxed, hands on thighs, looking straight forward. Take a slow breath in. (The young lady in the picture would be able to breathe more easily if she loosened or removed her belt.)

2. As you exhale, slowly drop your head on to your chest, concentrating on letting go of any tightness in the back of your neck.

3. As you begin a slow inhalation, roll your head around to the right, looking forward, and gently pull your head down so that your right ear is as near to your right shoulder as possible. Don't worry about any creaks you might hear.

4. Still breathing in, roll you head gently around until your chin is pointing at the ceiling. Let your head fall backward as far as is comfortable and look up as you pause.

5. As you begin to breathe out, roll your head around to the left, again looking forward, and gently pull your head down so that your left ear is as near to your shoulder as possible.

6. As you complete the slow breath out, let your head roll around to the front so that your chin is again resting on your chest.

Roll two or three times to the right and an equal number to the left.

Shrug

1. Sit tall and upright with your head balanced on top of your spine and your shoulders and arms relaxed, hands on thighs, looking straight forward.

2. As you begin a slow breath in, push your shoulders forward as far as you can.

3. Still breathing in, raise your shoulders as high and as close to your ears as you can. Pause, continuing to pull your shoulders upward.

4. As you begin to exhale, firmly pull your shoulders back, still keeping your arms relaxed.

5. As you complete the slow breath out, relax your shoulders, letting them fall downward and forward to the starting position.

Repeat two or three times.

Twist on a chair

1. Sit tall and upright on the front half of your chair with your shoulders and arms relaxed, hands on thighs, looking straight forward. Take a slow breath in.

2. As you begin to breathe out, slowly turn your chest, then your neck and your eyes to the right, making sure your pelvis does not twist on the seat. Move your left hand on to your right thigh, and reach behind you with your right hand to grasp the left edge of your seat. As you pause at the end of exhalation, help the twist by pulling gently with your hands.

3. As you inhale, slowly turn your chest, then your head and your eyes to the front again.

4. Repeat the twist on the other side.

Do three or four complete repetitions.

Back bend on a chair

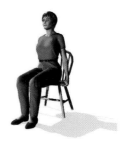

1. Sit tall and upright on the front half of your chair and hold the sides of your seat just behind your hips. Take a slow breath in.

2. As you exhale, bend your body backward, push your chest upward and forward, let your head fall back, look up and gently pull your shoulders downward with your hands. Keep up the tension as you pause.

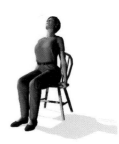

3. As you inhale slowly, release the tension and slowly return to the starting position, relaxing you shoulders.

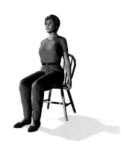

Repeat two or three times.

If you wish, you can then counter the back bends by exhaling as you bend forward in your seat, let your head flop and let your arms hang down so that your fingers rest on the floor near your feet. Take a few normal breaths in this position before slowly inhaling as you sit upright again.

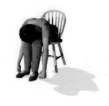

△ *Warning.* It is unwise to try this exercise on an office chair with wheels.

Ankle and knee bend

1. Sit upright well back in your chair and hold the edge of the seat near your hips.

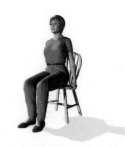

2. While taking a slow breath in, raise your right leg straight out in front of you and rotate your foot so that the toes make three or four clockwise circles.

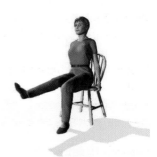

3. As you exhale, slowly bring your knee as high as you can towards your chest, grasp just below your knee with both hands and pull gently but firmly. Keep up the pull as you pause.

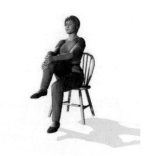

4. As you inhale, hold the sides of the seat again, straighten your leg, and rotate your foot so that the toes make three or four circles in an anticlockwise direction this time.

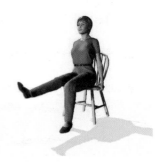

5. As you exhale, slowly lower your leg to the floor.

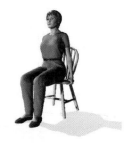

Repeat on the other side and do two or three complete repetitions.

△ *Warning*. It is unwise to try this exercise on an office chair with wheels.

Long distance travel: If you remain seated for a long time, for example while travelling on a long distance bus or train or during a long haul aeroplane flight, your inactive leg muscles no longer help to return blood to the heart and the pressure in veins in your legs increases. Fluid leaks into the tissues and your ankles tend to swell. Prolonged inactivity increases the risk that blood in the deep leg veins will clot (deep vein thrombosis). To reduce the risk of a blood clot, your doctor might recommend taking an aspirin with the last meal before leaving to 'thin' the blood. Try to drink plenty of fluids during the journey. Non-alcoholic drinks are best because alcoholic drinks increase dehydration.

Whenever you have the opportunity, get up and walk about. If you can stand but not walk about, keep raising your heels from the floor to contract your calf muscles. When seated regularly lift each foot from the floor and rotate it first one way and then the other as described above in the *Ankle and knee bend*.

Dynamic tension

This is another name for isometric exercise – the contraction of muscles without movement. It is a form of resistance training that can be used when any movement of the limbs is very difficult, for example, while sitting or standing on a crowded bus or underground train. It helps to increase muscle tone and strength but not flexibility.

1. Take a slow breath in.

2. As you slowly breathe out, do any of the following without moving:

   a. Contract the muscles of your shoulders as though you were trying to move them forward and pull them back at the same time

   b. Press both your hands down very strongly on your knees

   c. Tighten the muscles of your pelvic floor as though you had a desperate need to go to the lavatory and to pass water

   d. Contract the muscles of your thighs as though you were trying to kick you feet forward and pull them back at the same time

    e. Push you knees strongly against each other

    f. Press you toes strongly into the floor

You can contract any other sets of muscles you like. Keep up the tension as you pause for a few seconds.

3. Completely relax the tension as you breathe in again.

SECTION 4: EXERCISE, DIET AND HEALTH

Chapter 13: Exercise options for full fitness

Aerobic exercise *versus* strength training

There are two main kinds of exercise, aerobic exercise and strength or resistance training. In aerobic exercise little force is applied but there is a lot of movement. It is called aerobic because the relatively weak and short-lived muscular contractions have little effect on the muscles' blood supply, so oxygen delivery is unaffected. Some examples are walking, jogging, cycling and swimming. In strength training force is applied with relatively little movement, in the same way that sustained muscular contractions are used in *Slow Yoga*. It is sometimes called anaerobic exercise because the powerful contraction of muscles reduces their blood supply by squeezing the blood vessels, and so temporarily reduces the oxygen available to them. Much of the apparatus in fitness centres and health clubs is provided for strength training. Digging the garden, pushing a lawnmower, ironing and carrying shopping are more commonplace examples of the same kind of exercise. Aerobic exercise increases endurance with little effect on muscle strength, but strength training increases both strength and endurance because it also increases the body's capacity for aerobic exercise (p 20). Many training programs, sports, athletics and everyday activities use a combination of the two kinds of exercise

For complete fitness the most important muscle in your body, the heart, needs to be strengthened by regular aerobic exercise that is sufficiently intense to increase the heart rate and to cause some breathlessness. This provides a cardiac reserve that can be called on when unaccustomed aerobic effort is needed. The aerobic component of some popular exercise programs are discussed below.

Yoga

The oldest known evidence of Yoga practice dates back to about 2500 BC. The man responsible for Yoga's modern renaissance was Tirumalai Krishnamacharya. He was born in 1888, and after years of study established a school of Yoga in the palace of the Maharajah of Mysore where he taught from 1933 to 1955. He was over 100 when he died in 1989. He taught the founders of three of the four major schools of Yoga that are currently practised in the West. Recent books from each of the schools are listed on page 95.

Krishnamacharya's son, TKV Desikachar, gave up his job as an engineer in Denmark in 1962 to study with his father. He developed *Viniyoga*, a gentle, flowing form of Yoga that coordinates breathing with movement. Exercises are tailored to the individual. (*Slow Yoga* is based on the sequential exercises and coordinated breathing of Desikachar's *Viniyoga* with the addition of elements of strength training.) Krishnamacharya's brother-in-law, BKS Iyengar, developed *Iyengar Yoga*. It focuses on static poses and balance rather than flowing exercises, and makes much use of props such as belts and blocks. Another of Krishnamacharya's students, K Pattabhi Jois, devised *Astanga Yoga*, which involves a powerful workout. Vishnu Devananda founded the fourth school, *Sivananda Yoga*, which concentrates on 12 basic postures with variations and on proper breathing, exercise, diet, relaxation and 'positive thinking'. Devananda was sent to San Francisco in 1957 by his gurū HH Sivananda to spread Yoga teaching through the USA.

The Yoga renaissance that had been initiated by Krishnamacharya was brought to the West by his three students and by V Devananda, helped by the work being done in the USA by Richard Hittleman. He was born in New York in 1927, the son of a conservative Jewish family, and began to learn Yoga when he was only nine from the Hindu maintenance man at their family home in the Catskills. After studying Yoga in India he returned to Florida and established a Yoga school in 1957. His television series 'Yoga for Health', first shown in Los Angeles in1961 and later across North America and Europe, stimulated a wide interest in Yoga.

Of all the varieties of Yoga, only *Astanga Yoga* and its Western version *Power Yoga* provide aerobic exercise. It is very strenuous and makes one sweat. It is unsuitable for those who are unfit or out of condition. It has another potential drawback: while all the other forms of Yoga can be continued into old age, it seems unlikely that this would be possible with *Power Yoga*.

Pilates

German-born Joseph Pilates, while interned during the First World War, devised a method of body conditioning to help fellow internees regain their strength. It uses spring-controlled resistance to muscular contraction and so provides a form of anaerobic strength training. (Recently, the name Pilates has been inappropriately applied to floor-based exercises without the use of machines.) Like *Slow Yoga*, Pilates concentrates strength training on the core postural muscles of the spine and on the breathing muscles. The use of apparatus for strength training, whether in a Pilates studio, a fitness centre or a health club develops strength but does little to improve balance or flexibility. It does not involve aerobic exercise.

T'ai Chi

In the early morning in China groups practise the ancient art of *T'ai Chi* together in the open air. It was developed as a self-defence system based on yielding to the hand or foot attack of an aggressor and then, at the right moment and with minimum effort, pushing, locking or throwing the opponent. The term *T'ai Chi* refers to the symbol shown in the picture (called Yin and Yang), which illustrates the harmonisation of opposites - in yielding, there is strength.

The first record of a form of *T'ai Chi* familiar to present day practitioners dates from the 18th century in the Henan province of China. The modern shortened form was developed during the 1940s by Cheng Men-ch'ing, Professor of Painting in the Shanghai School of Fine Art. Following the communist take-over of China in 1949 he moved to Taiwan where he taught his new form of *T'ai Chi* as well as painting and calligraphy. When he moved to New York in 1964 he attracted many students who have since spread his teachings through North America and Europe.

The modern form of *T'ai Chi* emphasises the importance of breathing with the diaphragm, relaxation and self-awareness. Individuals make a series of slow movements of the hands and legs similar to the footwork and the thrust and parry of the arms used in the martial arts from which it originated. The slow movements of the limbs help to improve balance and posture and provide some measure of strength training. *T'ai Chi* is always performed standing up and it takes the joints of the spine and limbs through a narrower range of movement than Yoga, so somewhat less flexibility is developed. Recent research has shown that the regular practice of *T'ai Chi* by older adults has favourable effects on the heart rate and blood pressure as well as on balance. However, it does not provide aerobic exercise.

Choice of aerobics

We have seen that neither the practice of Yoga of any school except *Power Yoga* nor *T'ai Chi* nor the use of body building apparatus whether in a Pilates studio, a fitness centre or a health club provides the aerobic exercise that is needed to keep the heart healthy.

Suitable outdoor aerobic activities include brisk walking, jogging, distance running, cycling and taking part in sports or athletics. Aerobic activities that are not affected by bad weather include heavy housework, skipping, dancing, swimming, aerobics classes, and the use of exercise bicycles, rowing machines, steppers and treadmills.

△ *Warning*. Before starting an unfamiliar aerobic activity it would be wise to consult your doctor
- If you are under regular medical care for any reason
- If you get pain in the chest or arm when you exert yourself
- If you become more breathless than you had expected
- If you feel dizzy, faint or have palpitations during or after exertion.

Strolling is not an aerobic exercise, but taking a brisk walk with one or more companions is a pleasant way of combining aerobic exercise with social activity. Walking on rough ground or uphill is better than walking on the flat. When you take a step, let your heel reach the ground first, roll through the step from heel to toe, push the back leg forward with your toes using your calf muscles, then swing your pelvis to help the leg move forward. Do not stride too far in front of your body. If you place your hand in the small of your back, you should feel strong contractions of the erector spinae muscles on each side alternately.

For full fitness *Slow Yoga* sessions lasting 20-40 minutes on five or more days a week could be combined with three or more weekly sessions of any enjoyable aerobic exercise that lasts at least 20 minutes. Recent research has shown that repeated short aerobic sessions are as effective as less frequent long ones, so aerobic activity could be enjoyed in shorter sessions that total one or two hours a week.

Alternatively, instead of setting aside specific times totalling one or two hours a week for aerobic activity, you could alter your lifestyle: get off your bus or tube a stop early; park your car further from work; always use the stairs instead of the lift or escalator; walk down the corridor instead of telephoning; take a brisk walk at lunch time. Any activity that increases your pulse and makes you slightly breathless counts, even sex.

Chapter 14: Mutual benefits of exercise and a healthy diet

The medical profession has long accepted that aerobic exercise is good for your health. Only in the last few years have the health benefits of strength training of the sort used in *Slow Yoga* been recognised. This chapter describes how exercise and a healthy diet complement each other to reduce the risk of some serious medical conditions, and explains how strength training does this just as well as aerobic exercise.

Raised blood pressure

Exercise: Raised blood pressure increases the risk of stroke, heart failure and kidney disease. Blood pressure is conventionally measured twice: when the heart is contracting (systolic blood pressure) and when it is at its lowest between heart beats (diastolic blood pressure). Both aerobic exercise and strength training result in a significant reduction of resting systolic and diastolic blood pressure in normal people and in patients with raised blood pressure (systolic and/or diastolic hypertension). Strength training, but not aerobic exercise, also lessens the increase in blood pressure and heart rate that results from lifting and carrying heavy objects. Slow breathing exercises like *Slow breath lying* (p 12) have been shown to lower both systolic and diastolic blood pressure in patients with uncomplicated hypertension.

Diet: Reducing the amounts of fat and salt (sodium) in the diet reduces both systolic and diastolic blood pressure. It has been recommended that patients who have non-life threatening hypertension should be given advice about exercise and diet, and then should have their blood pressure measured regularly for four to six months before drug treatment is considered: it may not be needed. There is a case for all of us to reduce the high sodium content of our normal Western diets. We could eat less processed food that contains 'hidden' salt and add less salt to our food, perhaps using a salt substitute containing potassium as well as sodium at the table and in cooking.

Coronary heart disease

Exercise: Fat is carried in the blood stream combined with proteins. There are three main forms - chylomicrons, which appear in the blood after eating and carry fat from the intestine to the liver, and low- and high-density lipoproteins that are present in the blood even when fasting. The lipoproteins are measured by the cholesterol they carry. Low-density lipoprotein cholesterol is called 'bad' cholesterol because raised levels are associated with deposition of fat in arteries, and with an increased incidence of coronary heart disease and heart attacks. High-density lipoprotein cholesterol is called 'good' cholesterol because the lipoprotein helps to carry fat back from the tissues to the liver to be broken down and tends to clear blood vessels. Both aerobic exercise and strength training reduce fasting blood levels of 'bad' cholesterol and increase levels of 'good' cholesterol. In a large group of people with no history of heart disease and no symptoms, researchers found that in one year there were three times as many fatal heart attacks in those who took no exercise at all as in those who practised either moderate intensity aerobic exercise or strength training.

Diet: A Mediterranean diet has favourable effects on the lipoproteins, raising 'good' cholesterol and lowering 'bad' cholesterol. The diet is rich in the antioxidants beta-carotene, vitamin C, vitamin E and selenium that protect high-density lipoprotein from being broken down. It consists of eating more carbohydrate in which glucose is complexed into larger molecules like starch (bread, oats and potatoes, for example), more pulses, root vegetables and green vegetables, more fruit and more fish (particularly oily fish like herrings, sardines, mackerel, salmon, trout and tuna) but less meat, with a preference for poultry, and less sugar and fat. Margarine made from rapeseed oil and olive oil can be used instead of butter and the same oils can be used for salad dressings. Vegetarians need not despair that they are unable to benefit from the polyunsaturated fatty acids present in oily fish; those in rapeseed and olive oil have a similar effect in preventing heart attacks. Milk and yoghurt should be low fat, and the consumption of fried foods, cakes, biscuits, pastry products and chocolate must be reduced. The Mediterranean diet has been shown to reduce the frequency of heart attacks even in those who have suffered one before.

Those who take a couple of small alcoholic drinks a day have increased levels of 'good' cholesterol and a lower risk of heart disease than teetotallers. However, moderation is critical. More than four small drinks a day for men and three for women can increase 'bad' cholesterol, raise blood pressure and harm the liver. 'Binge' drinking is particularly harmful. The evidence that red wine is better for the heart than other kinds of alcohol remains controversial, though widely acclaimed. Interestingly, Japanese scientists found that people who drank moderately had higher IQs than teetotallers, whether they drank beer, whisky, wine or sake. However, drinking does not necessarily increase IQ – perhaps more of those with higher IQs knew about the effect of moderate drinking in reducing the risk of heart disease.

Major reasons for giving up smoking are that it seriously increases the risk of heart attacks, strokes and chronic lung disease as well as lung cancer (and probably colon cancer). Those hoping to start a family have an additional reason to stop smoking - men are likely to be less fertile and women have a reduced chance of conceiving, even if they are only passively exposed to smoke. When you decide you really want to give up, you may find that the *Slow breath* (p 6) will bring relief when you have unpleasant physical symptoms of nicotine withdrawal in the first month or so, and will also help to control irritability.

Obesity and diabetes

Exercise: If your body has a high ratio of fat to total weight you are at risk of developing diabetes, hypertension, osteoarthritis and coronary heart disease. In 1999 nearly one half of men and over one third of women in the UK were overweight.

When food intake is unchanged, aerobic exercise helps to reduce fat as a proportion of body weight by burning calories at the time the exercise is taken and for a short while afterwards. Strength training also reduces fat as a proportion of body weight by burning calories during exercise, but it has an additional effect because it increases muscle tone and, particularly in men, muscle mass. Larger muscles with better tone increase basal metabolic rate so that more calories are also burned at rest.

Adult onset (Type 2) diabetes is being increasingly diagnosed in Western societies, most commonly in people who are middle-aged or older, are sedentary and are obese. The patients have an acquired resistance to the action of insulin in the tissues, and as a result have increased blood glucose concentrations. Both aerobic exercise and strength training decrease raise fasting insulin levels, decrease the insulin response to glucose in the diet and decrease the resistance of tissues to the action of insulin. Only those muscles that have been exercised show decreased tissue resistance, so a comprehensive training program like *Slow Yoga* that involves most muscles is preferable to one like jogging that uses a more limited range of muscles. Reducing excessive body fat stores decreases the probability that Type 2 diabetes will develop, and is a major objective in its treatment. Doctors looking after diabetics who take up regular exercise often find that their patients' drug treatment needs to be reduced to prevent low blood glucose levels.

Diet: Attempting to reduce your calorie intake is a notoriously unreliable and usually temporary way of reducing fat stores. The encouragingly large amount of weight that can be lost in the first week or two after restricting food is almost all water that was bound up with glucose stores in the liver. The body then switches down its basal metabolism when food becomes short, so weight loss slows dramatically. Unless the calorie restriction is accompanied by strength training, muscle is lost as well as fat. Hunger develops with an intense urge to overeat. It is not surprising that the vast majority of those on a restricted diet are unable to maintain a low calorie intake for very long. 'Yo-yo' dieting is potentially dangerous – it has recently been found to lower the blood level of 'good' cholesterol.

The best advice is not to concentrate primarily on trying to reduce *how much* you eat, but to change permanently *when* you eat, *how* you eat and *what* you eat.

- *When to eat*: if circumstances allow, wait until you become really peckish before eating
- *How to eat*: concentrate your attention on the process of eating, on the food and on its taste, and stop when you have had just enough to satisfy your hunger. Don't try to work, read or watch television at the same time. Never feel guilty about not clearing your plate
- *What to eat*: the food in a Mediterranean diet (p 79) is bulky so it takes longer to eat and produces a sensation of fullness earlier than refined or processed food. Sweet foods, sweets, chocolates, and sugary drinks must be avoided unless they form a small part of a full meal. Taken on an empty stomach they raise blood glucose rapidly and stimulate insulin production. The insulin pushes down the high glucose level so that it is followed within an hour or two by a trough that produces an intense feeling of hunger. The carbohydrates in a Mediterranean diet are complex. They take longer for the body to break down to glucose, so swings in blood glucose levels after eating are flattened and there is no hunger trough.

Colon cancer

Exercise: Epidemiological surveys of large groups of people have shown that regular physical activity is associated with a decreased risk of colon cancer. There is a strong association with the amount of energy expended, sedentary people having the highest risk and those who take regular light, moderate or vigorous exercise increasingly lower risks. There is no clear distinction between the effects of exercise that is largely aerobic and exercise that primarily increases strength.

Diet: The risk of colon cancer is highest in those whose diet is rich in fat and meat. There has been conflicting reports about whether a diet high in fibre lowers the risk, negative studies having been of relatively short duration. However, epidemiological evidence points to the risk being lowest in those taking a diet rich in fruit and lightly cooked vegetables – a Mediterranean diet again.

Falls

Exercise: The elderly, particularly if they are frail with poor muscular development, are susceptible to falls. Strength training reduces the likelihood of falls particularly if, as in *Slow Yoga*, it is combined with exercises that improve balance. Aerobic exercise alone has little effect on strength and so does little to reduce the incidence of falls.

Diet: There are no dietary measures that will have a positive effect on muscle strength, but a low calorie intake can have a negative effect because it causes loss of muscle unless it is accompanied by regular strength training. Vitamin D deficiency, due either to inadequate dietary intake or to lack of exposure to sunlight, also has a negative effect: it causes weakness that affects the larger muscle groups, making it difficult to rise from a chair or to climb stairs. It is sometimes accompanied by muscle pains and cramps.

At one time anabolic steroids - the performance-enhancing drugs now banned in athletic competitions – were recommended for increasing muscle strength and bulk in wasted patients. They are dangerous whether taken by the young or the elderly. Side effects include acne and baldness, unstable and aggressive behaviour, failure of the testes with impotence and sterility and severe liver damage. Graded strength training is effective and much safer.

Fractures

Exercise: Osteoporosis (a weak bone structure) greatly increases the risk of fracture of the hip, spine and wrist. The density of bone usually reaches its maximum by the age of about 30. Maximum bone strength tends to be lower in those who take little exercise after puberty. It is uncertain whether the gradual fall in bone density after thirty is due to 'ageing' itself or to decreased physical activity. There is an accelerated rate of fall in women after the menopause unless they receive hormone replacement therapy. Bone needs the regular pull of muscle to maintain its normal structure. If osteoporosis has developed, the good news is that at all ages and in both sexes strength training and moderate weight-bearing aerobic exercise like brisk walking both prevent further bone loss and can even reverse it.

Diet: Maximum bone density is lower in those who have had a low calcium diet, particularly if it was associated with an inadequate intake of vitamin D or inadequate exposure to sunlight. Dieting to lose weight often reduces the amount of calcium-rich foods such as milk, cheese and bread that are eaten, and drinking diet colas containing phosphoric acid can interfere with calcium balance. Both increase the risk of osteoporosis. Young women who take excessive aerobic exercise, for example in athletics, aerobics or dance classes, and combine it with a low calorie diet run the risk of menstrual disturbances in the short term and of osteoporosis in the longer term. The beneficial effects of strength training and moderate weight-bearing aerobic exercise on osteoporosis are complemented by the calcium and vitamin D content of a Mediterranean diet. A word of warning: diets high in protein and salt cause loss of calcium from bone.

Failing memory

Exercise: A study of previously sedentary adults aged 60 to 75 years showed that those who were randomly assigned to a program of walking for 45 minutes three times a week showed a significant improvement in memory. In another study, normally active elderly people undertook a program of strength training similar to that used in *Slow Yoga* for eight weeks. At the end of the period there were improvements in both strength and memory. Remarkably, the memory effect was still present one year later. Recent research has shown that the brain is not as doomed to failure as had been thought, and that memory loss with age is not inevitable. The good news is that the brain can develop as we mature, making new cells with new connections. The process is stimulated by learning, experience and particularly by interaction with others. As well as continuing to exercise, we would do well to maintain our social contacts, our interest in new ideas and news, and stretch our minds with things like crossword puzzles, chess and creative activities. Use it or lose it!

Diet: To study anecdotal reports linking memory loss with tooth loss, Japanese research workers extracted the molar teeth from half of a group of mice so that they could eat but not chew. When they were young, mice with and without molars were equally good at finding their way through a maze. However, while older mice with molars were almost as good as young mice, those without molars could not remember the way. Studies of their brains showed deterioration of cells linked with short term memory, strongly suggesting that chewing helps to maintain memory. However, the suggestion that these mouse experiments prove that we should all either adopt the chewable unrefined Mediterranean diet or chew gum should be taken with a grain of salt.

Chapter 15: Exercises for some health problems

These exercises for eyestrain, neck, shoulder and arm pain, wrist and hand pain, low back pain, knee pain, urinary incontinence, constipation and catarrh may be worth trying to see if they help. However, if you are already under medical care for any of these conditions, ask your doctor for advice first.

Eyestrain

Prolonged office work, particularly if it involves concentrating on a computer screen, can cause aching or sore eyes. You can exercise the muscles inside the eye that alter the focus of the lens by occasionally looking into the distance for the period of a slow breath in and then back at your desk or screen as you breathe out. Repeat this change of focus three or four times. Three of the 'office' exercises in Chapter 12, the *Neck roll* (p 69), *Twist on a chair* (p 70) and *Back bend on a chair* (p 71), use the eye muscles and can make your eyes feel less tired.

If you wear bifocals you may find that your eyes and neck are much more comfortable with a pair of single focus glasses specifically prescribed for the distance between your eyes and the desk or monitor screen.

Eyes can be soothed and relaxed by the warmth and darkness of *Palming*. Rub your palms together vigorously until they become warm from the friction, then cover your closed eyes with your overlapping cupped hands so that the palms do not touch your eyelids. Hold the position for three or four slow breaths.

Neck, shoulder and arm pain

The commonest cause of neck, shoulder or arm discomfort or pain is a stooped posture. The weight of your head is no longer balanced on top of your spine but supported by neck muscles. Your shoulders are hunched and the curves of your spine in the upper part of your chest and neck region are exaggerated, narrowing the spinal nerve windows. Earlier in this book it was explained how you could find out if you have a permanently stooped posture, and some exercises that might improve things were suggested (p 18). Your muscle tone will improve and help you to achieve a normal posture if you adopt a regular *Slow Yoga* exercise plan and always try to think tall, sit tall and stand tall.

Symptoms can result from sitting with a curved back looking down at a desk or a badly placed computer screen for long periods. A particular danger is using a laptop computer actually on your lap because it becomes impossible to maintain a correct sitting posture. The laptop should be placed on a table at waist height and the keyboard used like that of a conventional computer.

When working at a desk or computer workstation, adjust the height of your seat so that when you sit tall with your upper arms relaxed, your elbows are at desk level.

Your thighs should be horizontal with no pressure behind your knees – use a footrest if necessary. The top of the monitor screen should be at eye level, and the desk should be positioned so that you cannot see reflections from windows or lights in the screen. (In the picture, the shadows show that light is coming from the wrong direction; the desk should be turned through ninety degrees.) Do not hold a telephone between your shoulder and your head.

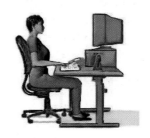

As we get older, creaking, cracking and grinding noises in the neck become increasingly common, sometimes associated with neck, shoulder and arm pain. This is usually called osteoarthritis of the neck joints. (Arthritis means joint inflammation, but the signs of inflammation – redness, swelling and heat – are rarely present. Rest and drugs are used to treat active arthritis with inflammation.) There is increasing research evidence that osteoarthritis without inflammation benefits if the affected joints are mobilised and the surrounding muscles strengthened.

Four of the 'office' exercises in Chapter 12 are particularly useful for relieving neck, shoulder and arm pain whether it is caused by bad posture or by osteoarthritis of the neck: the *Shrug* (p 69), *Neck roll* (p 69), *Twist on a chair* (p 70) and *Back bend on a chair* (p 71).

Stress can also induce neck, shoulder and back pain, often accompanied by 'tension' headache, caused by sustained muscular tension. Ways of coping with stress and its effects are discussed in the next chapter (p 91).

Localised shoulder pain

The shoulder is a complex joint. The head of the upper arm bone, the humerus, is held in position against the end of the collar bone (clavicle) and part of the shoulder blade (scapula) by muscles and their tendons as well as by ligaments. The tendons run in synovial sheaths and the muscles are separated from underlying tissues by small sacs of synovial fluid called bursas. Inflammation of a tendon sheath (tendonitis) or a bursa (bursitis) can produce localised shoulder pain which is often felt only when the arm is in a certain position, for example raised straight up. Tenderness is usually localised to a small area. The inflammation can follow the repeated lifting of a weight, often with difficulty and from a height, or from impact injuries. The pain usually responds to rest, but it can become chronic, particularly if the shoulder is rested too long. The first line of treatment (before embarking on injections of hydrocortisone or even an operation) is to mobilise the joint and strengthen the surrounding muscles. This is also the first line of treatment for the similar pain sometimes associated with osteoarthritis of the shoulder joint.

Several *Slow Yoga* exercises that use arm movements can be helpful: *Slow breath and stretch* (p 8), *Back arch standing* (p 22), *Forward and backward bend standing* (p 28), *Side pull standing* (p 37), *Twist standing* (p 42), *Forward bend and twist standing* (p 45), *Sideways bend and twist standing* (p 46), *Hand clasp* (p 48) and *Wrist and finger extension* (see below). The arm movements should never be taken so far as to produce pain, but should be pushed slowly and gently just to the edge of discomfort.

Until things improve it would be wise to avoid those exercises in which much of the weight of the body is carried by the shoulder joints: the harder version of *Forward and backward bend on hands and knees* (p 30), *Forward and backward bend on hands and feet* (p 30), *Forward bend and back arch* (p 32) and *All fours* (p 51).

Wrist and hand pain

Pain in the wrist and hand is often due to repeating the same activity for prolonged periods, for example, writing, typing, stamping forms or even knitting. This is sometimes called repetitive strain injury. The best way to avoid pain and discomfort is to take mini-breaks from the repetitive activity – say half a minute every five minutes or so. This is far more effective than longer breaks at longer intervals.

If you work at a desk, do not rest your wrist on the desktop when using a mouse or a keyboard so as to avoid damage to the tendon sheaths in the front of your wrist and to the median nerve. Try to let your wrists float above the desktop. When typing, move your hands by moving your upper arm from the shoulder so that you can reach all the keys easily without stretching your fingers forward or moving your wrists sideways.

Finger flexion This exercise helps to relieve aching in the fingers that can follow a prolonged session of writing or typing.

1. Place the tip of the index finger of the right hand on the back of the left hand just above the knuckle of the little finger, and with the thumb of the right hand gently push the little fingernail towards the knuckle. Hold for a few seconds.

2. Shift the thumb to the second joint of the left little finger and push it down towards the palm in the same way. Hold for a few seconds.

Repeat with all the fingers of the left hand and then repeat with all the fingers of the right hand. Finally, push the nail of each thumb towards the palm.

Wrist and finger extension This exercise incorporates two of the movements used in a successful trial of Yoga-based intervention for carpal tunnel syndrome that was published in the *Journal of the American Medical Association* in 1998. It is hoped that exercises like these will prevent the full syndrome developing. The exercise described below certainly eases wrist and hand discomfort caused by repeating the same activity for prolonged periods.

1. Sit tall and upright with your head 'balanced' on top of your spine and your shoulders and arms relaxed, hands on thighs, looking straight forward.

2. As you take a slow breath in, raise your elbows sideways and bring your hands together in front of your neck, fingers pointing upward. Press your palms firmly together, bending the wrists back as far as is comfortable. Pause for a few seconds.

3. As you breathe out, interlock your fingers and push your hands out in front of you, moving your shoulders forward.

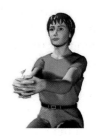

4. Still breathing out, turn your hands over so that the palms are facing forward. Straighten your elbows as you push your hands as far forward as is comfortable. Pause for a few seconds, keeping up the tension.

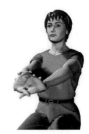

5. With your arms still straight, take a slow breath in as you raise you arms high above your head, pushing your hands upward. Pause for a few seconds.

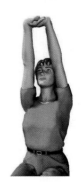

6. As you breathe out, lower your linked hands behind your head, keeping your elbows pulled back. Push forward against your head with your hands and push backward with your head to prevent any movement.

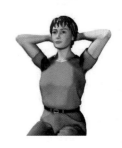

Repeat two or three times.

Low back pain

Back pain results in more absence from work in Western society than any other illness. It is most commonly caused by muscle, ligament or facet joint injury that results in spasm of the surrounding muscles and pressure on the spinal nerves. Other causes of low back discomfort or pain include a swayback posture with an exaggerated lumbar curve, perhaps caused by leaning back to counteract the increased abdominal weight of obesity or pregnancy, and side-to side bending from taking one's weight on one leg or sitting awkwardly for prolonged periods. A true 'slipped' disc with persistent pain in the buttock and down the leg is a relatively rare cause.

There is a natural tendency to rest the injured part. Although this may be necessary for a day or so, there is now no doubt that the best treatment for localised back pain is to return to activities that require spinal movement. To prevent recurrence both the spinal and the abdominal muscles must be strengthened and any abnormality of posture corrected. A daily program of *Slow Yoga* exercises is one way of achieving all these objectives. The 'shaving' exercises in Chapter 11 (p 65) make a gentle starting point, and can be done several times each day in the early stages, taking care not to push the movements to the point where they become painful or intensify an existing dull ache. Be particularly careful if you are taking an analgesic drug like paracetamol or ibuprofen. Subsequent strengthening of the spinal and abdominal muscles will require a commitment to daily programs of the kind suggested in Chapter 10 (p 53). A brisk daily walk is of value in helping to relieve spasm.

Reject the idea promoted by some orthopaedic mattress manufacturers that you need a hard bed. Your mattress should be sufficiently soft to accommodate your hip when you lie on your side so that your spine is not bent to one side, and to accommodate your buttocks when you lie on your back so that the normal lumbar curve is maintained.

PARTIAL HARD NESS O.K.

Knee pain

By far the commonest cause of chronic knee pain is osteoarthritis. It is a disease that becomes increasingly common with age. However, the condition can develop in early middle age in those who have suffered recurrent knee injuries in their youth, for example some former professional footballers, and in those who are overweight.

There is now good evidence from a randomised controlled trial that home exercises to strengthen the thigh muscles that flex and extend the leg reduce pain and improve function. Some *Slow Yoga* exercises that strengthen these muscles without using a great deal of force are *Back arch lying* (p 23), *Forward and backward bend sitting* (p 33), *Side raise lying* (p 41), *Twist lying* (p 44), and *Ankle and knee bend* (p 72).

More intensive weight-bearing exercises such as *Squat* (p 48) and *All fours* (p 51) should be deferred until pain and function have improved.

Knee rotation. The following exercise, which comes from traditional Chinese medicine rather than Yoga, is a gentle way of improving the mobility of your knee joints (and the ankle joints) and of increasing the strength of the muscles around your knees.

1. Stand with your feet two or three inches apart. As you exhale, lean forward, place your hands on your knees and bend your knees until your arms are vertical.

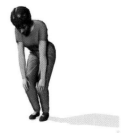

2. As you begin a slow breath in, rotate your hands and knees clockwise as far as is comfortable. Make sure that the soles of your feet remain in contact with the floor.

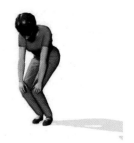

3. Still inhaling, continue to rotate and straighten your knees. Pause in full inspiration.

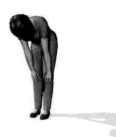

4. As you begin to exhale, continue to rotate your knees clockwise. Again make sure that the soles of your feet remain in contact with the floor.

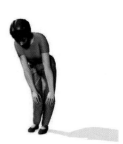

5. Still exhaling, bring you knees forward to the starting position and pause.

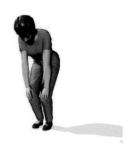

Rotate your knees three to six times clockwise and then an equal number anticlockwise.

Urinary incontinence

Leakage of urine on coughing, sneezing or laughing – stress incontinence – is a distressing complaint that is experienced most often by women who have had children. It can even start during pregnancy before the birth of a first child. The good news is that the condition can usually be greatly improved or cured by strength training of the muscles of the pelvic floor. These are the groups of muscles that prevent accidents when one has diarrhoea or a full bladder and that contract during orgasm. A recent trial of pelvic floor exercises for stress incontinence using eight to twelve contractions three times a day found that, after six months, more than half the women who took part considered that they no longer had a problem.

Slow Yoga exercises that strengthen the pelvic floor are *Forward and backward bend on hands and knees* (p 30) and *Pelvic tilt* (p 65). Pelvic floor contractions can be carried out independently of these exercises, but are best synchronised with the exhalation of a slow breath to ensure that each is held firmly for a sufficiently long time.

Constipation

Constipation is uncommon in those who eat a diet rich in unrefined cereals, pulses, root vegetables, green vegetables and fruit. However dehydration, for example after a long haul flight, can cause constipation whatever the diet. A change of routine like going on holiday affects some people. BKS Iyengar wrote that constipation can be cured by the effect of gravity on the bowel in the *Shoulder stand* (p 9). The following exercise can also be effective.

Abdominal lift During this exercise the contents of your abdomen are subjected to strong negative and positive pressures. It is possible that it relieves constipation by stimulating secretion of mucus by the glands in the wall of the large intestine and by stimulating contraction of the muscle of the bowel wall.

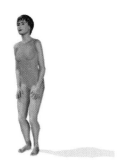

1. Stand with your knees slightly bent, bend forward a little and place your hands on the front of your thighs. Take a slow breath in, pause and then breathe out completely.

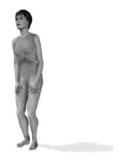

2. While still holding your breath, expand your chest as though you are trying to breathe in, letting your abdominal wall be sucked in as your diaphragm rises.

3. Still holding your breath, 'snap' your abdominal wall forward again, suck it back and repeat rapidly up to ten times. Then take a deep slow breath and relax, breathing normally.

This can be repeated five to ten times.

Catarrh, blocked ear tubes

A small tube (the Eustachian tube) runs between each inner ear and the back of your nose. Its function is to equalise the air pressure on each side of the eardrum. If a tube is blocked, your hearing can become muffled. A blocked tube can produce very severe pain in the ear if there is a big change in outside air pressure. Sweets are often offered on aircraft before take off because swallowing may help to clear a blockage and prevent pain when cabin pressure falls. The following Yoga exercise helps to clear catarrh from the back of the nose and to open the Eustachian tubes if they are blocked.

The Lion. During this breathing exercise, your tongue is protruded strongly to open the inner ends of the Eustachian tubes. Your eyes are opened wide and your gaze directed upward to stimulate the formation of tears which run into the nose through the tear ducts that start at the inner ends of your lower eyelids. (Tears contain an enzyme, lysozyme, that can help to kill bacteria.) In the full exercise your hands are pressed on your knees, providing strength training for your triceps and forearm muscles, but this is optional.

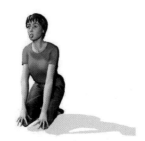

1. Kneel on the floor and sit on your heels. Press the palms of your hands firmly on your knees with the fingers spread wide. Open your eyes wide and look upward, keeping your head still.

2. Protrude your tongue as far as you can and, keeping your eyes wide open, take several slow breaths in and out through your nose until you feel your eyes fill with tears. (You would probably prefer not to do this exercise in a public place.)

3. Withdraw your tongue, release the hand pressure, sniff and swallow, breathing normally.

Repeat from step 1. A noise in both ears as you breathe in and out like the roaring of a lion indicates that the Eustachian tubes are clear.

Chapter 16: Managing stress

Good responses to stress

An airline pilot facing a potential disaster acts decisively to avert it. He is not aware of the automatic responses his body makes to help him react quickly and correctly. The moment the alarm signals reached his brain, endocrine glands are instructed to release two key hormones. Adrenaline primes his nervous system and increases his alertness, dilates his pupils, shunts blood from his gastrointestinal tract to his muscles, increases his pulse and respiration, raises his blood pressure and, together with cortisol which is secreted at the same time, raises the glucose level in his blood so that he is prepared for instant action. The Canadian doctor Hans Selye described these changes as the 'flight or fight' response to stress.

When the adrenaline and cortisol are flowing and positive physical action is being taken the stress response can be exhilarating. There is some evidence that a burst of cortisol affects the neurotransmitters dopamine and serotonin, producing euphoria in the same way as 'recreational' drugs. Some even seek the thrills that stress can produce by engaging in such activities as parachuting, bungee jumping and white-water canoeing. Sufficient stress to produce a little anxiety and tension before acting or speaking in public can add to performance. A positive response to the stress of a deadline can help it to be achieved rather than being missed because of mental paralysis.

Bad responses to stress

Stress has bad effects when it persists for a long time, particularly if a physical response is not possible. Some common causes at work are competitive working conditions, job dissatisfaction, a sense of stagnation and unfair work pressure. Other potential causes of continuing stress include bereavement, unresolved problems with family or colleagues, forthcoming examinations and even moving house. One major cause of stress that is often overlooked is inadequate sleep. As well as causing drowsiness, inability to think clearly, lack of concentration and impairment of the ability to learn, inadequate sleep induces stress.

Symptoms produced by chronic stress include headache and neck, shoulder and back pain due to sustained muscular tension. Sustained elevation of adrenaline and cortisol levels can produce digestive disturbances, including gastric ulcers. A continuous increase in cortisol leads to declining T-cell counts, an impaired immune response and susceptibility to colds and other infections. It also impairs the function of a part of the brain responsible for new learning and recall, and increases blood pressure. The blood levels of 'bad' cholesterol may be increased. Some of the psychological effects of chronic stress are restlessness, irritability, anger, anxiety and depression. These can lead to 'comfort eating' and obesity, and to drug and alcohol abuse. Stress often has a detrimental effect on interpersonal relationships, and can cause loss of libido, impotence and insomnia.

Some pre-existing diseases are exacerbated by stress. These include raised blood pressure, diabetes, coronary heart disease, gastrointestinal problems, asthma, skin complaints and allergies.

Coping with stress

If you are able do something about removing the cause of your stress, do it. Concentrate solely on the cause rather than on your reaction to it. Some people seem to be able to do this far better than others, and respond to stress as a challenge and opportunity rather than as a hurdle or pressure. Try to have the courage to express your feelings and say what you are feeling rather than harbouring unhappiness, worry or silent resentment - doing so is likely to have much less serious consequences than those resulting from chronic stress itself. Discuss the problem with your partner, your colleagues or your boss. If you can, sort out disagreements and be prepared to take criticism. If your colleagues at work are not supportive, you should seriously consider changing your job for the sake of your health. Smoking, drinking too much and eating when you are not hungry may seem to help, but in the long term will make things worse.

One way that may help to reduce stress at work is by prioritising tasks (make a list) rather than trying to 'multitask' like a computer. To complete a single task efficiently in an office situation, turn off the phone and bleep, forget faxes and emails and make it clear that interruptions are unwelcome. Try not to take on more than you can deal with. If unfair demands are being made on you, say so.

Yoga offers two ways to help cope with stress – exercise and alert relaxation.

Exercise: There is a large body of research showing that exercise reduces the effects of stress, relieves depression and anxiety, improves mood and self-esteem, and gives more restful sleep. The US Surgeon General's report 'Physical Activity and Health' (p 95) emphasises that to obtain these beneficial effects light exercise needs to be taken on most days of the week. Both aerobic exercise and strength training of the kind used in *Slow Yoga* have been shown to be effective.

A *Slow Yoga* session first thing in the morning will help you to cope with the stresses of the day, and perhaps another short session before your evening meal may help you wind down. The exercises in Chapter 12 (p 69) can be used during the day in the office or while travelling to help relieve the aches, pains, stiffness and muscular tension caused by stress.

Alert relaxation: If stress can cause disease then it is reasonable to believe that peace and calm can improve health. People who are distressed are often advised to sit down, take a deep breath and relax. There is no doubt that slow deep breathing relaxes purposeless muscular tension and calms an overactive mind. A recent investigation showed that, while conventional relaxation exercises made volunteers sleepy and sluggish, relaxation exercises with concentration on Yoga-type slow deep breathing, on releasing muscular tension and on self-awareness had a markedly invigorating effect on feelings of physical and mental energy, and greatly increased positive mood. The fundamental difference is that during Yoga relaxation one remains alert. Alert relaxation is also part of *T'ai Chi*. The oldest surviving medical text, *Huang Di Nei Jing* (The Yellow Emperor's Canon of Internal Medicine), written in the second century BC, says that to remain free of disease 'one must breathe the vital energy (*Chi*) by concentrating one's mind and relaxing one's muscles'.

One of the breathing exercises in Chapter 2, the *Slow breath lying* (p 12) , describes how to combine attention to slow breathing with attention to muscle relaxation.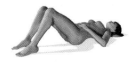

 Throughout this book I have used phrases like 'Breathe slowly, concentrate on what you are doing and feeling, and don't let your mind wander'. Past memories, future plans and associated ideas will enter consciousness; attention must be directed back to the present moment, the exercise and the sensations. Live in the present. As in every day life, worrying about the past and anxiously planning for the future can exacerbate stress and always detracts from the pleasure of the moment.

In *Slow Yoga* awareness of breathing and of sensations produced by the exercises need concentrated attention. Single-minded attention is a valuable facility for problem-solving, and is invaluable for improving skills in games and sports. Wimbledon champions and World chess champions both possess the facility. It has been proposed that alert single-minded concentration of attention during complete muscular relaxation is a useful working definition of meditation. It is probably not the sort of thing Patañjali intended when he wrote about meditation in the *Yoga Sūtra*, but it has even helped to improve the competitive performance of both a basketball team and a rifle shooting team.

ENVOI

'The young, the old, the extremely aged, even the sick and
the infirm obtain perfection in Yoga by constant practice...
Constant practice alone is the means of success.'

Haṭha Yoga Pradīpikā

FURTHER READING

Anatomy and physiology of exercise

Anatomy and Human Movement: Structure and Function (3rd edition). N Palastanga, D Field, R Soames. Butterworth Heinemann, Oxford 1998.

Exercise physiology (2nd edition). WD McArdle, FI Katch, VL Katch. Lea & Febiger, Philadelphia 1986.

Scientific Basis of Athletic Conditioning (3rd edition). AG Fisher, CR Jensen. Lea & Febiger, Philadelphia 1989

The Physiological Basis for Exercise and Sport (5th edition). EL Fox, RW Bowers, ML Foss. WCB Brown & Benchmark, Madison 1993

Importance of maximal resistance training. AC Guyton, JE Hall. In *Human Physiology and Mechanisms of Disease* (6th edition). Saunders, Philadelphia 1997; 692-3.

Schools of Hatha Yoga popular in the West

Iyengar Yoga
Light on Yoga. BKS Iyengar. Thorsons, London 2001.

Power Yoga
Power Yoga: the Total Strength and Flexibility Workout. BB Birch. Fireside Books, New York 1995.

Sivananda Yoga
The New Book of Yoga. Sivananda Yoga Centre. Ebury Press, London 2000.

Viniyoga
The Heart of Yoga: Developing a Personal Practice (2nd edition). TKV Desikachar. Inner Traditions International, Rochester 1999.

A comprehensive American list of Yoga resources which includes some web sites and addresses of organisations outside the USA is given in *Yoga for Dummies* by G Fuerstein and L Payne. IDG Books Worldwide, Foster City 1999.

Exercise and health: comprehensive research reviews

Physical Activity and Health: a Report of the Surgeon General. US Department of Health and Human Services, National Center for Chronic Disease Prevention and Health Promotion, 1996. This excellent report and summaries of its key messages for the general public are available as Adobe Acrobat files from the Chronic Disease Center web site: http://www.cdc.gov/nccdphp/sgr/sgr.htm

Benefits and Hazards of Exercise. Ed. D. MacAuley. BMJ Books, London 1999. Each chapter is written by research workers of international repute in the field and the book covers the most important aspects of exercise medicine.

Exercise and health: research review articles

Colon cancer
Does physical activity prevent cancer? Evidence suggest protection against colon cancer and probably breast cancer. D Batty. *BMJ* 2000; **321**: 1424-5.

Diabetes
Prevention of type 2 diabetes. KMV Narayan, BA Bowman, ME Engelgau. BMJ 2001; **323**: 63-4.

Frailty
Exercise and physical activity for older adults. American College of Sports Medicine. *Med Sci Sports Exerc* 1998; **30**: 992-1008.

Heart disease
Resistance exercise in individuals with and without cardiovascular disease. Committee on Exercise, Rehabilitation and Prevention, Council on Clinical Cardiology, American Heart Association. *Circulation* 2000; **101**: 828-33.

Exercise prescription in heart disease. CA Speed, LM Shapiro. *Lancet* 2000; **356**: 1208-10.

Immunity
Exercise and the immune system: regulation, integration and adaptation. BK Pedersen, L Hoffman-Goetz. *Physiol Rev* 2000; **80**: 1055-81.

Mental health
Physical activity and mental health: current concepts. SA Paluska, TL Schwenk. *Sports Med* 2000; **29**: 167-80.

Obesity
Resistance training and energy balance. ET Poehlman, C Melby. *Internat J Sports Med* 1998; **8**: 143-59.

Osteoarthritis
Medical management of osteoarthritis. K Walker-Bone, K Javaid, N Arden, C Cooper. *BMJ* 2000; **321**: 936-40.

Osteoporosis
The effect of progressive resistance training on bone density: a review. JE Layne, ME Nelson. *Med Sci Sports Exerc* 1999; **31**: 25-30.

Effects of lifestyle interventions on bone health. RW Keen. *Lancet* 1999; **354**: 1923-4.

Pregnancy
Exercise during pregnancy: a clinical update. JF Clapp. *Clin Sports Med* 2000; **19**: 273-86.

Urinary incontinence
Management of urinary incontinence in women. R Thakar, S Stanton. *BMJ* 2000; **321**: 1326-31.

Exercise and health: research reports

Carpal tunnel syndrome
Yoga-based intervention for carpal tunnel syndrome: a randomized trial. MS Garfinkel, A Singhai, WA Katz *et al. JAMA* 1998; **280**: 1601-3.

Failing memory
The effects of resistance training on well-being and memory in elderly volunteers. P Perrig-Chiello, WJ Perrig, R Ehrsam *et al. Age Ageing* 1998; **27**: 469-75.

Heart failure
Yoga and chemoreflex response to hypoxia and hypercapnia. L. Spicuzza, A Gabutti, C Porta *et al. Lancet* 2000; **356**:1495-6. (Editor's correction: *Lancet* 2000; **356**: 1612.)

Raised blood pressure
Walking to work and the risk of hypertension in men: the Osaka health survey. T Hayashi, K Tsumura, C Suematsu *et al. Ann Intern Med* 1999; **130**: 21-6.

Low back pain
Randomised controlled trial of exercise for low back pain: clinical outcomes, costs and preferences. JK Moffett, D Torgerson, S Bell-Syer *et al. BMJ* 1999; **319**: 279-83.

Osteoarthritis
Evaluation of a Yoga based regimen for treatment of osteoarthritis of the hands. MS Garfinkel, HR Schumacher, A Husain *et al. J Rheumatol* 1994; **21**: 2341-3.

A randomized trial comparing aerobic exercise and resistance exercise with a health education program in older adults with knee osteoarthritis. WH Ettinger, R Burns, SP Messier *et al. JAMA* 1997; **277**: 64-6.

The effectiveness of exercise therapy in patients with osteoarthritis of the hip or knee: a randomized clinical trial. ME van Baar, J Dekker, RA Oostendorp *et al. J Rheumatol* 1998; **25**: 2432-9.

Effectiveness of home exercise on pain and disability from osteoarthritis of the knee: a randomised controlled trial. SC O'Reilly, KR Muir, M Doherty. *Ann Rheum Dis* 1999: **58**:15-9.

Pregnancy
Effects of aerobic and strength conditioning on pregnancy outcomes. DC Hall, DA Kaufmann. *Amer J Obstet Gynecol* 1987; **157**:1199-203.

Urinary incontinence
Single blind, randomised controlled trial of pelvic floor exercises, electrical stimulation, vaginal cones and no treatment in the management of genuine stress incontinence in women. K Bo, T Talseth, I Holme. *BMJ* 1999; **318**: 487-93.

INDEX